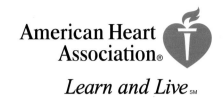
American Heart Association®

Learn and Live SM

Heartsaver First Aid

D1402643

Editor
Leon Chameides, MD

Contributing Editors
Tom P. Aufderheide, MD
Paul Berlin, MS, NREMT-P
Louis Gonzales, BS, NREMT-P
Mary Fran Hazinski, RN, MSN
Edward Stapleton, EMT-P
Albert L. Wyatt, Jr

Senior Science Editor
Mary Fran Hazinski, RN, MSN

Task Force on First Aid
Leon Chameides, MD, Chair
Tom P. Aufderheide, MD
Paul Berlin, MS, NREMT-P
Louis Gonzales, BS, NREMT-P
Mary Fran Hazinski, RN, MSN
Edward Stapleton, EMT-P
Albert L. Wyatt, Jr

Illustrator
Anne Jorunn Svalastog

**Task Force for
Evidence-Based First Aid —
*ECC Guidelines 2000***
Leon Chameides, MD, Chair
Paul Berlin, MS, NREMT-P
Richard O. Cummins, MD, MPH, MSc
Louis Gonzales, BS, NREMT-P
Judy Goodman
Mary Fran Hazinski, RN, MSN
Mark C. Henry, MD
Lenworth M. Jacobs, MD, MPH
Robb S. Rehberg, MS, ATC, NREMT
Donna Seger, MD
Adam Singer, MD
Edward Stapleton, EMT-P
Lark Stewart, MS, NREMT
David A. Zideman, MD

ISBN 0-87493-416-8

Contents

Preface

This student manual is part of the American Heart Association Heartsaver First Aid Course. This manual contains the 3 sections of *Heartsaver First Aid* that constitute the basic course—General Principles, Medical Emergencies, and Injury Emergencies—plus the section on Environmental Emergencies. We have tried to make the course practical and easy to understand by adhering to the following principles:

■ We did not try to be comprehensive. We limited ourselves to the emergencies that a first aid rescuer is *most likely* to encounter at the worksite.

■ We have included only the assessments and interventions that can be applied by a *trained lay rescuer* and that have been shown to make a difference.

■ We have avoided technical medical language in favor of language that a layperson can easily understand.

The Heartsaver First Aid Course is video-based and includes peer practice and case discussions. It has been extensively pilot-tested in the field. This manual includes many revisions based on the results of that testing. Although the first aid presented in this course can be used in any setting, the course was specifically designed for emergencies in the workplace.

The course was developed on the basis of evidence-based guidelines. Evidence-based guidelines are important because

■ The process determines the strength of the scientific evidence that supports the recommended first aid interventions. We have included only those assessments and interventions that have been shown to be effective.

■ The process includes a built-in mechanism to periodically review and update the evidence.

This manual can be used as a text as well as a workbook. You will learn the material best if you read the manual before the course, use it as a workbook during the course, and then periodically use it as a reference and review guide.

Leon Chameides, MD

General Principles of First Aid

Chapter ①

First Aid: How Will It Help Me?

Case Example

Your company has asked you to learn how to give first aid. You are about to take a first aid course. As you get ready to take the course, some questions cross your mind:

- *What is first aid?*
- *Do I have to help? What is my responsibility?*
- *Will I get into legal trouble if I make a mistake?*
- *Will I remember what I have learned? Will I be able to act in an emergency?*

What You Will Learn

By the end of this chapter you should be able to

- Explain what first aid is
- Describe your responsibility and possible risk
- Know where to find a list of items in the First Aid Kit at your worksite

What Is First Aid?

First aid is the *immediate* care that you give to a victim of an illness or injury *before* professional medical rescuers arrive.

Your actions during the first minutes of an emergency can be critical. What *you* do may help a victim recover more completely or more quickly. Most of the time you will give first aid for minor illnesses or injuries. But you may also be called upon to give first aid for a serious illness or injury, such as a heart attack or major bleeding. The first aid that you provide may mean the difference between life and death. Or it may mean the difference between a quick recovery and a long period of disability. *You* can make a difference!

Do I Have to Help?

If you drive past a car crash, *you* can decide whether to stop and help. If you are walking down the street and see a person who seems ill, *you* can decide if you will help. The choice is *yours!*

But if giving first aid is part of your job description, you *must* help during your working hours. You may be assigned to give first aid in addition to your other work, or it may be part of your job description. Law enforcement officers, firefighters, flight attendants, lifeguards, and park rangers have a duty to give first aid as part of their job when they are working. But even they can decide whether to stop and help when they are off duty.

What Is My Responsibility? What Are My Risks?

You have a duty to give the level of care that you will learn in this first aid course. You have a legal responsibility to act the way a reasonable person with your level of training would act. No one expects you to give the level of care given by a professional such as an EMS rescuer, a nurse, a physician, or other healthcare worker.

Remember: A person who is ill or injured has the right to refuse care. If the victim is responsive, introduce yourself *before* you touch him/her: "My name is Joe Smith and I am trained in first aid. May I help you?"

- If the victim agrees, you may give first aid.
- If the victim refuses your help, phone your company's emergency response number (or 911), and stay with the victim until medical rescuers arrive.
- If the victim is confused or cannot answer, assume that he/she would want you to help.

Will I Remember What I Have Learned? Will I Be Able to Act in an Emergency?

This course will teach you how to recognize an emergency and what to do. But if you don't use or practice your skills often, you will forget them. We all forget things that we don't use often. To be prepared to help in a real emergency, you must learn the material and practice the skills. Then every 1 or 2 months you should review and practice what you have learned. Use this manual to help you review.

Critical Fact
Remember: **If you don't use it, you will forget it.**
Review and practice your skills often.

The First Aid Kit

The First Aid Kit contains supplies that you might need in an emergency. Keep the supplies in a sturdy container that is clearly labeled and water-resistant. You and anyone else who might need to use the kit must know where it is kept. Every time you use something from the kit, replace what you have used. Check the kit after each use to make sure it is complete and ready for another emergency.

Not all first aid kits contain the same supplies. Your company will decide what supplies the First Aid Kit should contain. The Appendix (on page 19) to this section lists a sample of supplies that might be useful in a First Aid Kit.

Chapter 2 — *Protect Yourself — Protect the Victim*

"Dead heroes can't save lives. Injured heroes are a nuisance. So check the scene for hazards before you lurch in."

— Nancy L. Caroline,
Emergency Care in the Streets

Case Example

A truck has struck an employee in the parking lot. You see a man lying on the ground. Several co-workers have gathered around him. You note that traffic is moving slowly around the crash.

Would you know what to do?

What You Will Learn

By the end of this chapter you should be able to

- Name 5 things you should look for at the scene of an injury

- Explain what "universal precautions" are

- List 2 diseases that universal precautions may prevent

- List 3 pieces of personal protective equipment

- Show the correct way to remove protective gloves

- Tell what you should do if you are exposed to blood or other body fluids

Scene Safety

You may have to give first aid in dangerous places. The victim may be in a room with poisonous fumes or on a busy street or a company parking lot. You and others near the victim(s) will be nervous and excited, especially if you know the victim. You will have to make important decisions. You may not be thinking about harm or injury to yourself.

Remember: *You must not put yourself in danger while trying to help others. You could become a victim when you are trying to be a rescuer. Always look around and check for safety—safety for yourself and safety for the victim!*

Always look around and make sure the area is safe for you and the victim. **Do not waste time.** Look around as you approach the victim (Figure 1).

What Are You Looking For?

As you approach the scene, you should think about the following:

- **Is there any danger for the rescuer?** Sometimes rescuers are injured while trying to provide first aid. Watch your footing. Watch where you are going. **Do not attempt a dangerous act!** Examples of acts that might be dangerous include crossing multiple lanes of a busy interstate highway or entering an area with spilled gasoline or downed power lines.

- **Is there any danger for the victim?** As a general rule, do not move an ill or injured victim.

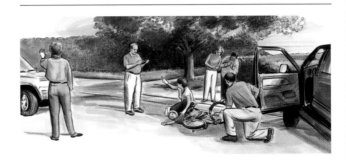

FIGURE 1. Ask others to direct traffic and phone your company's emergency response number.

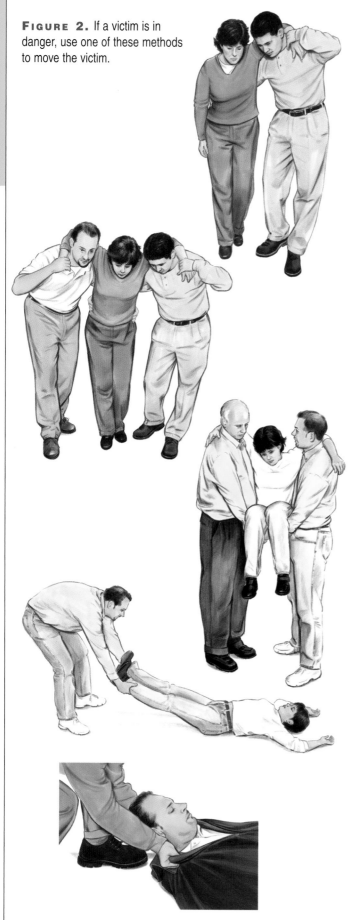

FIGURE 2. If a victim is in danger, use one of these methods to move the victim.

One of the few times you should move a victim is if the area is unsafe and poses a danger. If you do have to move the victim from danger, such as a fire or collapsing building, use one of the methods shown in Figure 2.

■ ***Are there other people around who can help?*** Ask others to direct traffic and phone your company's emergency response number (or 911). That way you can begin to give first aid to the victim (Figure 1).

■ ***How many people are injured? How were they injured?*** Look around to be sure you see everyone who might need help. Try to get an idea of what happened.

■ ***Where is the nearest telephone? Does anyone have a cellular phone?*** Ask someone to phone your company's emergency response number (or 911).

■ ***What is your location?*** Address, floor, location in building or on the property.

Protection From Blood-Borne Diseases

This section is based on recommendations of the Occupational Safety and Health Administration (OSHA).

Body fluids, such as blood, saliva, and urine, can sometimes carry germs that cause diseases.

Whenever you give first aid you should

■ Use personal protective equipment provided by your employer. Throughout this manual we will assume that you use personal protective equipment whenever the equipment is available. Personal protective equipment (Figure 3) includes

— Protective gloves, which you should wear whenever you give first aid

— Eye protection, which you should wear if a victim is bleeding

— Face mask or face shield, which you should use whenever you give rescue breaths

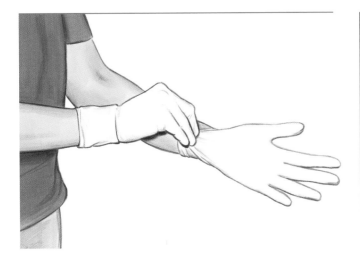

FYI...

Latex Allergies

Some rescuers and victims may be allergic to latex. So use protective gloves that don't contain latex whenever possible. For example, use vinyl gloves.

If you *or the victim* has a latex allergy, do *not* use gloves that contain latex.

If you have a latex allergy, notify your emergency response program supervisor and your Heartsaver First Aid instructor before taking the course.

FIGURE 3. Wear protective gloves whenever you give first aid and wear eye protection if a victim is bleeding.

- Place all disposable equipment that has touched body fluids in a biohazard waste bag and seal it (Figure 4). *Don't throw the biohazard waste bag in the trash.* Follow your company's plan for disposing of hazardous waste.

- Wash your hands *well* with soap and water after properly taking off your gloves (Figure 5).

These steps are called "universal precautions": *"Universal"* because you should treat *everyone* as if he/she were infected and *"precautions"* because they are intended to protect you and your co-workers.

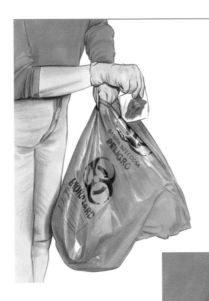

FIGURE 4. Place all disposable equipment that has touched body fluids in a biohazard waste bag and seal it.

If You Are Exposed to Blood or Body Fluids

If despite your best efforts you come in direct contact with blood or other body fluids, do the following:

1. If you are wearing gloves, take them off first. Use a paper towel to turn the faucet on and off and to push the soap dispenser button so that you don't leave germs. Immediately wash your hands and the contact area thoroughly with soap and water. Work up a lather for at least 15 seconds, and rinse your hands very well. Dry your hands with a paper towel. If you cannot wash immediately, clean your hands with a wet hand wipe and wash as soon as possible. If the victim's body fluids have splattered in your eyes, nose, or the inside of your mouth, rinse these areas thoroughly with water.

2. Tell your company's emergency response program supervisor what happened as soon as possible. Then contact your doctor.

Critical Facts

How to Take Off Protective Gloves

After you have given first aid, the outside of your gloves may have touched the victim's blood or other body fluids. So take your gloves off without touching the outside of the gloves with your bare hands. Here is how you do it (Figure 6):

■ Grip one glove on the *outside* of the glove near the cuff and peel it down until it comes off inside out. Cup it with your other (gloved) hand.

■ Place 2 fingers of your bare hand inside the cuff of the glove that is still on your hand.

■ Peel that glove off so that it comes off "inside out" with the first glove inside it.

■ Dispose of the gloves properly by putting them in a biohazard waste bag.

■ Wash your hands thoroughly with soap and water.

FYI...

Germs and Diseases

Blood-borne diseases are diseases caused by germs that may be present in the victim's blood or other body fluids. A rescuer can catch these blood-borne diseases if germs in an infected victim's blood or body fluids enter the rescuer's body. They might enter through the mouth, the eye, or a cut on the skin. To be safe, rescuers should wear personal protective equipment—gloves and eye shield (goggles)—to avoid touching the victim's blood or body fluids.

The most important blood-borne diseases are

■ Human immunodeficiency virus (HIV), the virus that causes AIDS

■ Hepatitis

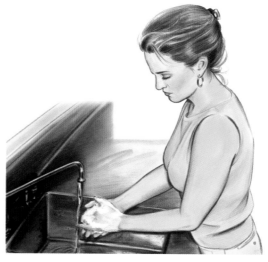

FIGURE 5. Wash your hands well with soap and water after properly taking off your gloves.

1.

2.

3.

4.

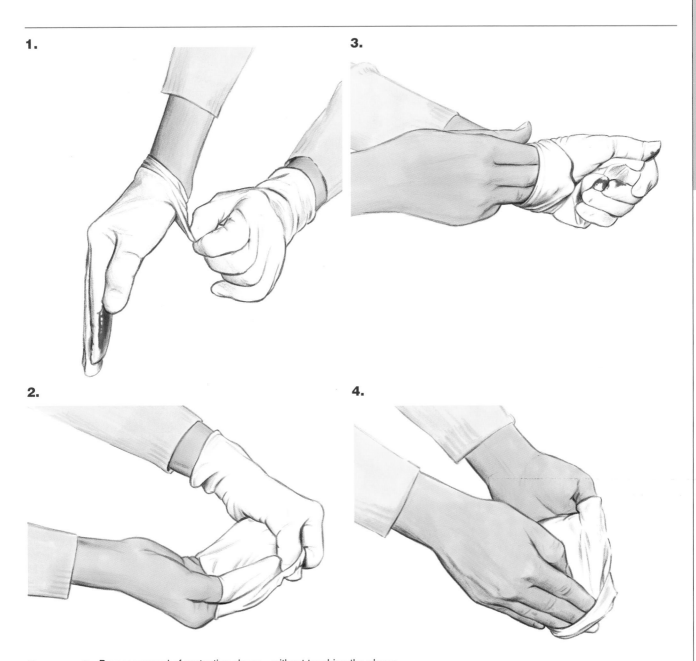

FIGURE 6. Proper removal of protective gloves—without touching the gloves.

Chapter 3

When in Doubt, Always Phone for Help

The AHA Chain of Survival

The American Heart Association adult Chain of Survival (Figure 7) shows the most important actions needed to treat life-threatening emergencies in adults. The first link in this adult Chain of Survival is to phone an emergency number to get help. This chapter will teach you how and when to phone.

What You Will Learn

By the end of this chapter you should be able to

- Tell how to phone your company's emergency response number

- Tell how to contact the EMS system in your area

- Give 5 examples of when you should phone your company's emergency response plan or 911 for help

Emergency Response Plan

Every place of business should have an emergency response plan (ERP). The emergency response plan tells workers *who, how,* and sometimes *when* to phone for help in an emergency.

How to Phone for Help

Your company's emergency response plan may be to call security, a response team, or the local EMS system number (in many communities 911). You should know your company's emergency response number and phone that number whenever you need help. Write the emergency response number in the Critical Facts box below, on a big sign in the First Aid Kit, and on a large sign near the telephone (Figure 8).

In many communities you can contact EMS by phoning 911. Find out what the number is in your community. If you don't know the number, phone "O" (operator). Some companies have emergency call buttons. If that button serves as the emergency response signal, you should know where it is located so that you can activate it in an emergency.

Critical Facts

Your Company's Emergency Response Telephone Number

If there is an emergency in this area, phone:

_____(fill in blank).

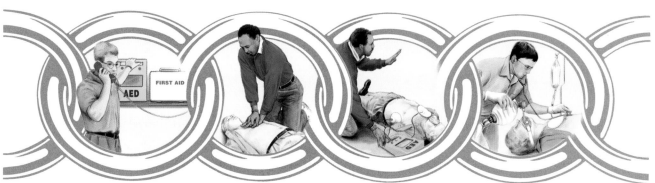

© 2002 American Heart Association

FIGURE 7. The AHA Adult Chain of Survival. The 4 links or actions in the chain are (1) phone for help, (2) begin CPR, (3) early AED use, and (4) transfer to advanced care.

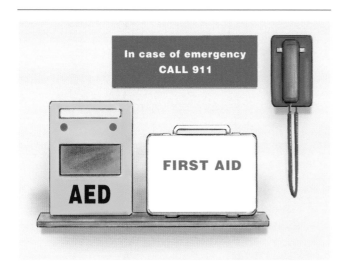

FIGURE 8. Write the emergency response phone number on a big sign in the First Aid Kit and on a large sign near the telephone.

When to Phone for Help

Your company may have specific instructions about when you should phone the emergency response number. In this manual we will tell you when to phone for help in specific emergencies. As a general rule, you should phone the emergency response number (or 911) and ask for help whenever someone is seriously ill or hurt or whenever you are not sure what to do.

If others are present, it is better to ask someone else to phone the emergency number and bring the First Aid Kit while you give first aid to the victim. If you are alone, shout for help while you begin to give first aid. If no one answers your shout, leave the victim to phone your company's emergency response number or 911. Phone for help, get the First Aid Kit, and return to the victim.

If you are not sure whether to phone your company's emergency response number, **do it!** It is better to phone for help even if you might not need it than not to phone when someone does need help!

Critical Facts

If You Are in Doubt, Phone the Emergency Number

When in doubt: phone your company's emergency response number or 911.

Critical Facts

When to Phone Your Company's Emergency Response Number or 911

Phone your company's emergency response number or 911 whenever someone is seriously ill or injured. Here are some examples.

- When you are not sure what to do
- If a victim is unresponsive
- If a victim has chest pain
- If a victim has a problem breathing
- If a victim has a severe injury or burn
- If a victim has a seizure
- If a victim suddenly can't move a part of the body (paralysis)
- If a victim has received an electric shock
- If a victim has been exposed to poison
- If a victim tries to commit suicide or is assaulted, regardless of the victim's condition

When you phone your company's emergency response number or the EMS operator, be prepared to answer some questions about the emergency. Here are some sample questions you may be asked and sample answers.

- **"What is your emergency?"**

  Sample answer: "A truck has hit an employee."

- **"How many people are injured?"**

  Sample answer: "One person."

- **"What number are you calling from?"**

    Sample answer: "The number here is 555-1313."

- **"Where is the victim located?"**

    Sample answer: "At the XYZ Company at 1234 Fifth Avenue. He is in the parking lot. Someone will meet you in the first driveway after you cross 3rd Street."

- **"What is happening now?"**

    Sample answer: "He is awake and bleeding from the leg. A first aid rescuer is trying to stop the bleeding."

Do not hang up until the dispatcher tells you to do so.

Case Example (continued)

At the beginning of the second chapter of this section, you read a short case example:

A truck has struck an employee in the parking lot. You see a man lying on the ground. Several co-workers have gathered around him. You note that traffic is moving slowly around the crash.

You read the following question: *Would you know what to do?*

Now you know what to do.

As you approach the victim, you quickly look around to see who is there and whether the area is safe for you and the victim. You tell one worker to stand in the road and direct all traffic away from the scene. You ask another worker to phone your company's emergency response number (or 911) and bring the First Aid Kit. You kneel beside the victim. He is breathing and responds to you. You say, "Hi, my name is Joe/Jane Smith, and I have training in first aid. We've phoned for help. May I help you?" The First Aid Kit arrives, and as you put on protective gloves, you note that the victim's leg is bleeding.

Chapter Before You Can Help, You Have to Know the Problem

What You Will Learn

By the end of this chapter you should be able to

- List 5 things you should look for in a victim (from the most important to least important)

- Describe how an unresponsive victim behaves

- Describe how a responsive victim behaves

- Show how to open the airway of an unresponsive victim

- Show how to check if a victim is breathing

- Tell how to look for bleeding

- Tell how to check for medical information jewelry

- Tell how to ask a responsive victim what the problem is

How to Find Out What the Problem Is

After you have made sure the area is safe, you have to find out what the problem is before you give first aid. Learn to look for problems in a certain order. First look for problems that may be life-threatening. The following steps will help you find out what the problem is. They are listed in order of importance, with the most important step listed first.

1. When you arrive at the scene, be sure it is safe to go to the victim. As you walk towards the victim, try to look for signs of the cause of the problem.

2. Check whether the victim is responsive. Shake the victim gently and shout, "Are you OK?" (Figure 9).

   - A victim who is *"responsive"* will respond in some way. But remember that a responsive victim may become unresponsive, so you have to keep on rechecking.

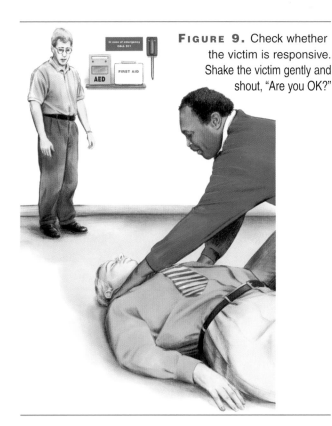

FIGURE 9. Check whether the victim is responsive. Shake the victim gently and shout, "Are you OK?"

- A responsive victim who is awake can answer your question. Introduce yourself, ask for permission to help, and ask the victim what the problem is.

- A responsive but very sleepy victim will only be able to move or just groan when you shake the victim and shout. Phone or ask someone to phone your company's emergency response number (or 911) and get the First Aid Kit.

- A victim who is *"unresponsive"* does not move or react in any way when you shake him/her. Phone or ask someone to phone your company's emergency response number (or 911) and get the First Aid Kit and AED if your company has one and you or a co-worker is expected to use it.

13

3. Next, look to see if the victim is breathing normally.

In a **responsive** victim who is *awake,* you can simply look to see if the victim is breathing normally. In a *responsive* but very *sleepy* victim, you may have to open the airway to check if the victim is breathing normally (see below).

If the victim is **unresponsive,** you have to open the airway before you can check whether the victim is breathing.

Open the airway with a head tilt–chin lift (Figures 10 and 11). Push down on the forehead gently with one hand and lift the chin with fingers of your other hand. If the victim has a head or neck injury, you will open the airway using a jaw thrust. You will learn this method in the section on Injury Emergencies.

FIGURE 10. Open the airway with a head tilt–chin lift.

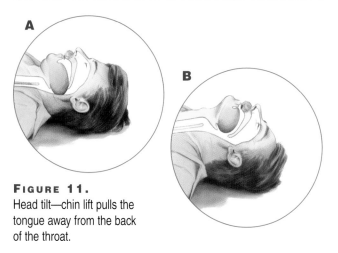

FIGURE 11. Head tilt—chin lift pulls the tongue away from the back of the throat.

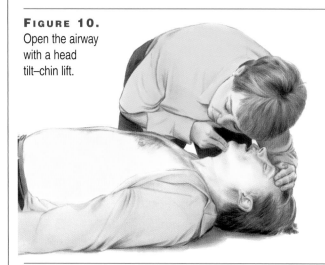

Now **check breathing.** Hold the airway open and place your ear next to the victim's mouth and nose. Look to see whether the chest is moving. Listen for breaths. Feel for breaths on your cheek.

4. Next, look for any obvious bleeding.

5. Finally, look for a medical information bracelet or necklace. It will tell you if the victim has a serious medical condition (Figure 12).

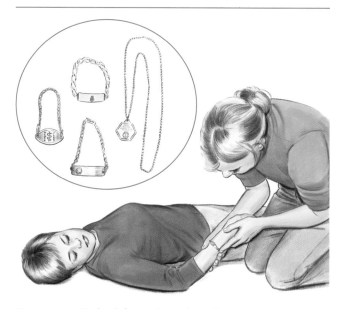

FIGURE 12. Look for medical information jewelry.

FYI...

Airway Obstruction in the Unresponsive Victim and the Responsive but Sleepy Victim

The muscles at the back of the throat relax in an unresponsive victim. They may also relax in a responsive but very sleepy victim. As a result, the tongue may fall back and block the airway. A victim with a blocked airway cannot breathe. Tilting the head back and lifting the chin forward pulls the tongue away from the back of the throat and opens the airway (Figure 11). You have to open the airway in an unresponsive victim before you can check whether the victim is breathing. You may have to open the airway in a responsive but sleepy victim.

FIGURE 13. Checking to See What the Problem Is.

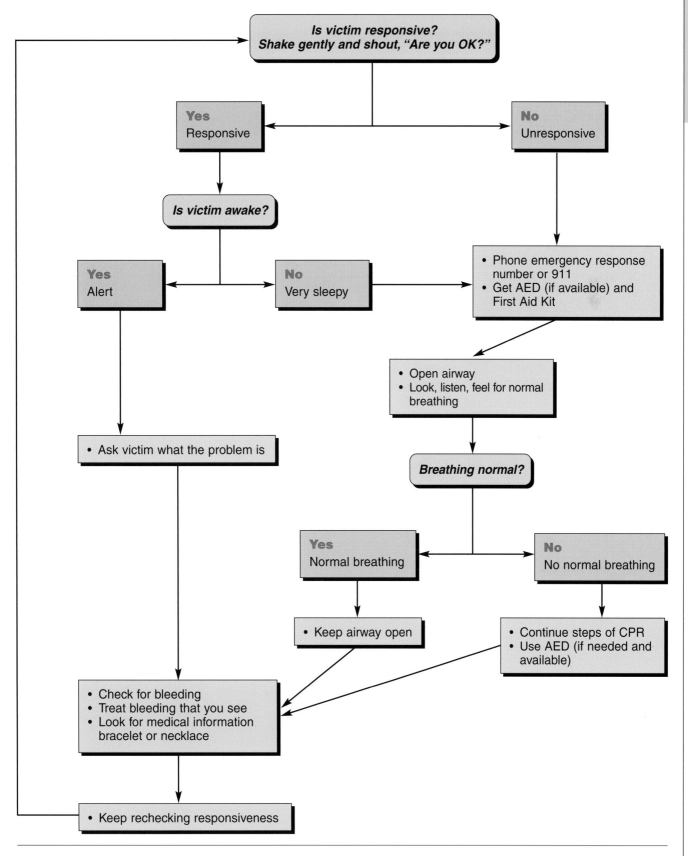

Chapter 5

After the Emergency Is Over

Case Example

You are giving first aid to a victim when EMS rescuers arrive and take over. You tell them what happened. They bring out a lot of equipment and work to save the victim. You stand on the side. EMS rescuers place the victim in an ambulance and drive away. As you fill out the forms required by your company, you begin to feel sad. The next day you find out that the victim died. You become anxious and can't get the emergency out of your mind. You constantly wonder whether you could have done something more.

What You Will Learn

By the end of this chapter you should be able to

- Tell how a first aid rescuer might feel after an emergency

- Tell which forms your company wants you to fill out after you give first aid

- Discuss the importance of *not* telling your co-workers private medical information that you might learn when you give first aid.

Medical Care for the Victim

As a first aid rescuer, you will not need to decide whether the victim needs further medical care after you have given first aid. The victim, workplace policy, or EMS rescuers in consultation with the victim will make that decision.

Emotions of the Rescuer

After the excitement of an emergency you may feel a "let down" if the outcome is good or bad. After all, during the initial moments of the crisis you had a lot of responsibility. As soon as others, such as EMS rescuers, take over, you may feel pushed aside, left out, and unappreciated. You may feel guilty and blame yourself if the outcome is not good. These feelings are common to all rescuers, no matter how experienced or knowledgeable they are. It is very important for you to be able to discuss these feelings with a counselor, doctor, nurse, or other healthcare provider.

Confidentiality

As a first aid rescuer you will learn private things about your co-workers, such as the medical condition. You must give all information about a victim to EMS rescuers and your company's emergency response program supervisor, but you must **not** share this information with other co-workers. Keep private things private (Figure 14).

Reporting

Your company may ask you to fill out a report after you have given first aid. If your company does not have a special report form, you might want to complete a form similar to the one in the Appendix to this section. Ask your supervisor if this form will meet your company's policy.

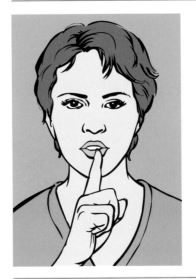

FIGURE 14. You must not share the victim's medical information with other co-workers.

Review Questions

1. Your company has asked you to take a first aid course and be responsible for providing first aid on your shift. What is first aid?

   a. The immediate first care given to a victim of an illness or injury before professional medical rescuers arrive

   b. The help given a new employee as orientation to a new job

   c. The medical care given to a victim of an illness or injury by professional medical rescuers

   d. Medical help given in a hospital or doctor's office

2. You are an assigned first aid rescuer. Which of the following phrases best describes your responsibility as a rescuer?

   a. Give first aid if you feel like it

   b. Give first aid when you are on duty

   c. Give the type of aid given by EMS rescuers

   d. Give aid even when the victim does not want it

3. You are a first aid rescuer. You are called to the scene of a car crash involving an injury at your workplace. Which of the following should you do *first*?

   a. Decide who is at fault

   b. Check that everyone has his/her insurance card

   c. Look around to make sure that the area is safe for you and the victim

   d. Call the police

4. You are a first aid rescuer. You have been asked to bring the First Aid Kit and give first aid to a co-worker who has been injured in the workplace. His arm is bleeding. Which of the following should you do?

   a. Before helping him, you put on personal protective equipment

   b. Put away the personal protective equipment because you do not need to wear it if you know your co-worker well

   c. After you have stopped the bleeding, you make sure to carefully throw all the blood-soaked bandages in the trash

   d. Do not touch anything until EMS personnel arrive

5. Which of the following is NOT a normal part of personal protective equipment used for first aid in the workplace?

   a. Gloves

   b. Eye shield

   c. Face mask or face shield for rescue breathing

   d. Shoe covers

6. Which of the following best describes your company's emergency response plan (ERP) for first aid rescuers?

   a. The ERP tells EMS rescuers where to go to help

   b. The ERP tells you, the first aid rescuer, whom to call for help, when to call for help, and how to call for help

   c. The ERP lets victims choose the hospital that they want to use for emergencies

   d. The ERP helps supervisors gather the proper reports for workplace emergencies

How did you do?

1. **The correct answer is a.** First aid is the immediate first care given to a victim of an illness or injury *before* professional medical rescuers arrive.

   Answer **b** is incorrect because first aid is taught only to carefully selected workers and is not given to employees as part of their general orientation.

   Answers **c** and **d** are incorrect because first aid is given by laypersons before trained medical rescuers arrive.

2. **The correct answer is b.** As an assigned first aid rescuer, your responsibility is to provide first aid when you are on duty.

   Answer **a** is incorrect because if you are on duty you must give first aid.

   Answer **c** is incorrect because you are expected to give the type of care described in this course. You are not required to give the type of care that a professional rescuer would give.

   Answer **d** is incorrect because if the victim is able, he/she must give you permission to give aid. If the victim does not want you to give aid, call and start your company's emergency response plan and stay with the victim until help arrives.

3. **The correct answer is c.** Whenever you approach a victim, always check the scene to make sure the area is safe for you and the victim.

   Answers **a, b,** and **d** are incorrect because a first aid rescuer does not have a responsibility to decide who is at fault, check insurance cards, or call the police before helping the victim.

4. **The correct answer is a.** You should always put on personal protective equipment before touching a victim's body fluids, such as blood.

   Answer **b** is incorrect because you should always wear personal protective equipment even if you know the victim well.

   Answer **c** is incorrect because you should not throw blood-soaked material in the trash. You should carefully dispose of it in a biohazard bag.

   Answer **d** is incorrect because you should try to provide care before the emergency medical services (EMS) personnel arrive.

5. **The correct answer is d.** Personal protective equipment *does not* include shoe covers.

   Answers **a, b,** and **c** are incorrect because personal protective equipment *does* include gloves, eye shield, and a face mask or face shield.

6. **The correct answer is b.** Your company's emergency response plan tells you, the rescuer, where you can get help when you need it, when to call for that help, and how to call for that help.

   Answer **a** is incorrect because the emergency response plan does not tell EMS where to send help. The person who calls the emergency response number must tell the dispatcher where to send help.

   Answer **c** is incorrect because the importance of the ERP is not in allowing a victim to select hospitals for care.

   Answer **d** is incorrect because the importance of the ERP is not to determine the paperwork that must be completed.

Appendix
Sample First Aid Kit

Description	Quantity
List of important local emergency telephone numbers, including police, fire department, EMS, and poison center	
Flashlight and extra batteries	1
Multipurpose scissors	1
Tweezers	1
Disposable gloves (small, medium, large, and extra large)	2 pairs in each size
Protective eye shield	1
Adhesive bandage strips	20
Sterile eye pads	2
Sterile gauze pads (4″×4″)	6
Sterile trauma pads (5″×9″)	2
Sterile trauma pads (8″×10″)	1
Roll of gauze (2″ wide)	3 rolls
Roll of gauze (4.5″ wide)	3 rolls
Adhesive tape (1″ to 2″ wide)	1 roll
Elastic roller bandage, 4″ and 6″ wide	1 roll of each
Sealed moist towelettes (hand wipes)	12
Emergency Mylar blanket	1
Face mask or face shield	2
Triangular bandages	2
Disposable instant-activating cold packs	2
Resealable plastic bags (quart size)	2
Biohazard waste bag (3.5 gallon capacity)	1

Appendix
Sample Medical Emergency Response Report

Date and time of report _____ Date and time of incident _____

Name of victim _____

Victim's employee no. _____ Location of emergency _____

Equipment involved in emergency _____

What was the victim's problem? _____

_____

Did the injury or illness involve any of the following? (Check all that apply.)

☐ CPR

☐ Automated external defibrillation
  (use of an AED)

☐ Breathing assistance

☐ Bleeding

☐ A fall

☐ An electric shock

☐ Burn

☐ Head

☐ Eye (R) (L)

☐ Arm (R) (L)

☐ Leg (R) (L)

☐ Hand (R) (L)

☐ Foot (R) (L)

☐ Poisoning

☐ Other

_____

_____

What happened?

_____

_____

_____

_____

List all responders who helped with the emergency

_____

_____

_____

What happened to the victim? _____

Name of person completing report _____

Date _____

Appendix
Practice Session

You will be having practice sessions during the course. You will be asked to refer to the following information.

Check Responsiveness and Phone the Emergency Response Number

In the practice session you will take turns being the victim, the rescuer, the bystander, and the dispatcher. You will get an opportunity to practice playing each role. The following directions will tell you what to do in each role.

Victim

- Lies down.
- Is not responsive.
- Checks to make sure that rescuer does all the steps in the right order as outlined below.
- Waits until rescuer has finished before correcting rescuer.

Rescuer

- Checks victim for responsiveness (victim is unresponsive).
- Tells bystander to phone the company emergency response number (or 911).
- Opens the airway using head tilt–chin lift.
- Looks, listens, and feels for breathing (victim is breathing).
- Checks for bleeding.
- Checks for medical information jewelry.

Bystander

- Phones the company emergency response number (or 911).
- Answers dispatcher's questions.

Dispatcher

Asks:

- "What is your emergency?"
- "How many people are injured?"
- "What number are you phoning from?"
- "Where is the victim located?"
- "What's happening now?"

Says:

- "An ambulance will be there. You may hang up now."

When the bystander and dispatcher have finished, they watch the rescuer and victim while waiting their turn.

Medical Emergencies

Chapter *You Have to Breathe to Live*

What You Will Learn

By the end of this chapter you should be able to

- Tell how to recognize someone with a breathing problem

- Describe the signs of choking

- Describe the first aid actions for a victim who is choking but can speak or make a sound

- Show the first aid actions for a victim who is choking and can't speak or make a sound

- List the signs of a bad allergic reaction

- List the first aid actions for someone with a bad allergic reaction

- Describe how you would use an epinephrine pen if your state regulations and company policy allow

Breathing Problems

Body cells need oxygen to work properly. When you breathe, air goes down the airways into the lungs (Figure 1). Oxygen then passes into the blood, which carries it to cells throughout the body. A person can't live without breathing. Anything that causes problems in breathing is an emergency.

The airways can suddenly become partly or completely blocked by

- The tongue falling to the back of the throat in an unresponsive or very sleepy victim

- Something, such as food, going down "the wrong way"

- Swelling of the lining of the airways, for example in a bad allergic reaction (Figure 2)

Breathing problems can also occur in victims with heart attacks, stroke, and some injuries.

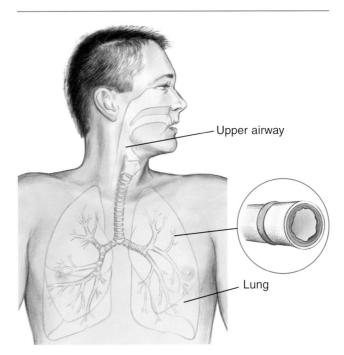

FIGURE 1. When you breathe, air goes down the airways into the lungs. Insert shows an open, small airway.

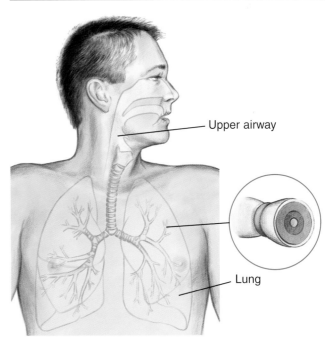

FIGURE 2. Swelling of the lining of the airways (see insert) can be caused by a bad allergic reaction or an asthma attack.

Signs of Breathing Problems

Breathing is normally so smooth and easy that we hardly notice it.

You can tell if someone is having trouble breathing if the person

- Is breathing very fast or very slowly

- Is working hard with every breath

- Has noisy breathing—you hear a sound or whistle as the air enters or leaves the lungs

- Has trouble making sounds or speaking more than a few words at a time

Many people with medical conditions, such as asthma, know about their condition and carry inhaler medicine that can make them feel better within minutes of using it (Figure 3).

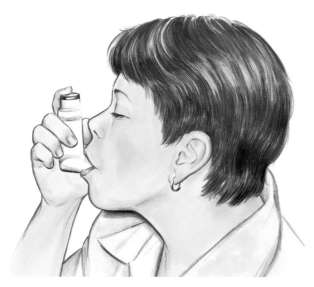

FIGURE 3. Many people with breathing problems carry inhaler medicines that can make them feel better within minutes.

Actions for Breathing Problems

If someone has trouble breathing:

1. Ask whether the victim has medicine and help get it.

2. Phone the company emergency response number (or 911) if

- The victim has no medicine

- The victim does not get better after using his/her medicine

- The victim's breathing gets worse, the victim has trouble speaking, or the victim becomes unresponsive

Choking

Case Example

You are eating lunch in the cafeteria. You hear loud voices at the next table. A man is grabbing his throat and is unable to breathe, speak, or make any sounds. He is very frightened. Several people are shouting at him. They don't know what to do.

Would you know what to do?

Signs of Choking

The most common cause of choking in adults is food that "goes down the wrong way" and blocks the windpipe.

If an object "goes down the wrong way" but does not block the windpipe completely, the victim will cough very hard and be able to make sounds.

If the windpipe is *completely* blocked, no air can enter. The victim can't breathe, talk, or make a sound. If this lasts more than a minute or so, the victim will become unresponsive.

A victim who has a completely blocked windpipe

- May grab his/her neck with one or both hands to tell you that he/she can't breathe (Figure 4)

- Is not able to speak or make sounds

- Cannot breathe

Actions for Choking

If the victim *can* breathe, cough, or speak, some air is getting into the lungs:

1. Be prepared to help but do *not* do anything.

2. Allow the victim to try to cough up whatever is blocking the windpipe.

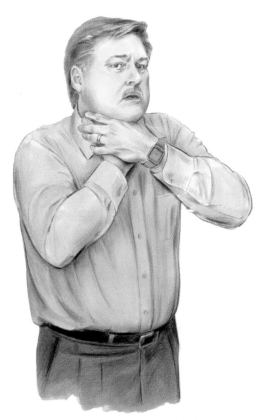

FIGURE 4. Universal choking sign (hands clutching the neck).

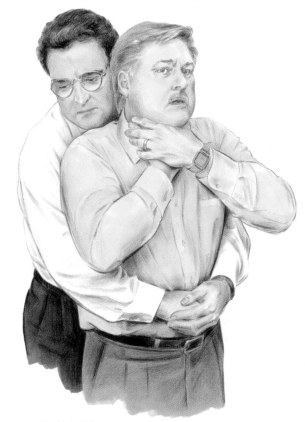

FIGURE 5. Heimlich maneuver.

If the victim *cannot* make sounds, cough, speak, or breathe, the windpipe is completely blocked:

1. Tell the victim that you are going to help and move behind the victim.

2. Provide abdominal thrusts (the Heimlich maneuver):

   - As you stand behind the victim, wrap your arms around his/her waist. Be sure that you are standing firmly with good balance, ready to help the victim down if the victim becomes unresponsive.

   - Make a fist with one hand.

   - Put the thumb side of the fist on the victim's abdomen, a little above the victim's belly button and well below the breastbone.

   - Grasp the fist with your other hand and push quickly upward and into the victim's abdomen (Figure 5).

- Repeat these quick pushes (thrusts) until
  - The object comes out of the victim's mouth or
  - The victim can breathe and make sounds or
  - The victim becomes unresponsive

If the victim is too large (for example, over-weight or pregnant) for you to wrap your arms around the waist, wrap your arms around the victim's chest and do chest thrusts instead of abdominal thrusts (Figure 6).

- If the victim becomes unresponsive:
  - Lower the victim to the floor.
  - Phone or ask someone to phone your company's emergency response number (or 911).
  - Begin the steps of CPR. When you open the victim's airway, look for the object blocking the windpipe. If you see it, try to remove it.

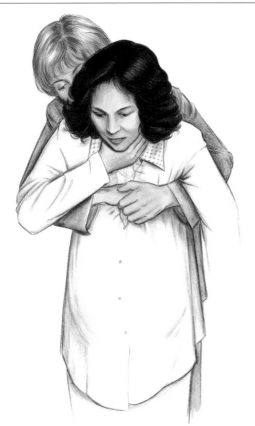

FIGURE 6. If the victim is too large for you to wrap your arms around the waist, wrap your arms around the victim's chest and do chest thrusts.

Case Example (continued)

At the beginning of this discussion of Choking, you read a Case Example:

You are eating lunch in the cafeteria. You hear loud voices at the next table. A man is grabbing his throat and is unable to breathe, speak, or make any sounds. He is very frightened. Several people are shouting at him. They don't know what to do.

You read this question: Would you know what to do?

Now you know what to do.

You ask the victim, "Are you choking?" He nods his head "yes." You ask, "Can you speak?" He shakes his head "no." You say, "I'm going to help you." You stand behind him, wrap your arms around his abdomen, and give several abdominal thrusts. A piece of meat flies out of his mouth. Now he can talk and breathe more easily. He thanks you.

Allergic Reactions

Case Example

At a company picnic a 38-year-old woman eats a cookie and complains that she is having trouble breathing. She tells you that she is very allergic to peanuts.

Would you know what to do?

Signs of Mild and Bad Allergic Reactions

Many allergic reactions are *mild,* but you should remember that *a mild allergic reaction could become a bad allergic reaction within minutes.*

A victim with a mild allergic reaction may have

■ A stuffy nose, sneezing, and itching around the eyes

■ Itching of the skin

■ Raised, red rash on the skin (Figure 7)

You will know that the reaction is a *bad* allergic reaction if the victim also has

■ Trouble breathing

■ Swelling of the tongue and face (Figure 8)

FYI...

Common Allergies

People can be allergic to many things, including

■ Many foods, such as

— Eggs

— Peanuts

— Chocolate

■ Insect stings or bites, especially bee stings

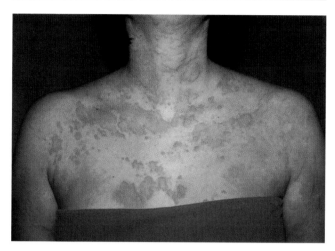

FIGURE 7. One sign of an allergic reaction can be a raised, red rash on the skin. Reprinted from *Principles and Practice of Dermatology,* Sams WM Jr, Lynch PJ, Figure 44-1, Copyright 1990, with permission from Elsevier Science.

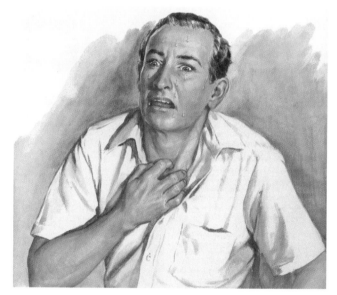

FIGURE 8. You will know if it is a bad allergic reaction if the victim has trouble breathing and if there is swelling of the tongue and face. Reprinted from *The Ciba Collection of Medical Illustrations,* Vol. 7: Respiratory System, with illustrations by Frank H. Netter, Divertie MB, editor, plate #120, Copyright 1980, with permission from Icon Learning Systems.

Actions for Bad Allergic Reactions

If you see signs of a *bad* allergic reaction, you should do the following:

1. Phone or ask someone to phone your company's emergency response number (or 911) and get the First Aid Kit.

2. If the victim is responsive and has an epineph-rine pen, ask the victim to use it. (An epineph-rine pen is also called an epinephrine injector.) Victims who carry epinephrine pens know when and how to use them. If the victim cannot give the injection, you may help if you are trained and approved to do so by your state regulations and by your company (see below).

3. If the victim becomes unresponsive, do CPR as needed.

4. If possible, save a sample of the substance that caused the reaction. This may be helpful if this is the victim's first allergic reaction.

Using the Epinephrine Pen

Some states and worksites permit first aid rescuers to help victims use their epinephrine pen (see the next page). Your instructor will tell you whether your state and worksite allow it.

Case Example (continued)

At the beginning of this discussion about Allergic Reactions, you read the following Case Example:

At a company picnic a 38-year-old woman eats a cookie and complains that she is having trouble breathing. She tells you that she is very allergic to peanuts.

You read this question: Would you know what to do?

Now you know what to do.

You ask a co-worker to phone your company's emergency response number (or 911) and get the First Aid Kit. You introduce yourself and ask for permission to help. You note that the victim is hav-ing trouble breathing. She is making high-pitched, noisy breathing sounds. She is pale and sweaty and has red blotches on her face, neck, and chest. She tells you that she has an epinephrine pen in her purse. You remove the epinephrine pen from the victim's purse and help her use it. She is start-ing to feel better by the time EMS rescuers arrive.

Critical Facts

How to Use an Epinephrine Pen

The epinephrine injection is given in the side of the thigh.

The steps for using an epinephrine pen are as follows:

1. Get the prescribed pen.

2. Take off the safety cap (Figure 9A). Follow the instructions printed on the wrapper.

3. Hold the injector in your fist without touching either end because the needle comes out of one end. Press the tip of the pen hard against the side of the victim's thigh, about halfway between the hip and knee, through clothing if necessary. Hold the pen in place for several seconds (Figure 9B).

4. After using the injector, follow your company's policy for "sharps" disposal or give the pen to the EMS rescuers for proper disposal.

5. Write down the time of the injection. This information may be important for the victim's care by EMS rescuers. You can write it on a piece of paper and later transfer the time of the injection to your report.

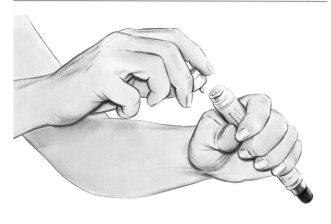

FIGURE 9A

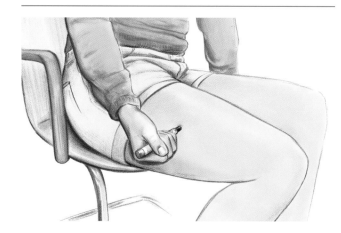

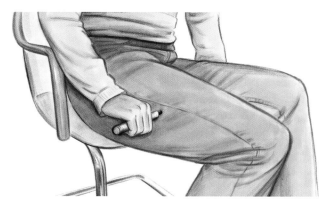

FIGURE 9B

Chapter **2** *Chest Pain and Heart Attack*

Case Example

A middle-aged co-worker complains that he has felt an uncomfortable pressure in his chest for the last 15 minutes. You introduce yourself and ask if you may help. You notice that he is short of breath.

Would you know what to do?

What You Will Learn

By the end of this chapter you should be able to

- List several words that a victim of a heart attack may use to describe the pain or pressure caused by a heart attack

- Describe where the pain or pressure of a heart attack might be located

- Describe first aid actions for a victim with chest pain or pressure

Signs of a Heart Attack

Signs of a heart attack may include

- **An uncomfortable feeling in the center of the chest that lasts for more than a few minutes**

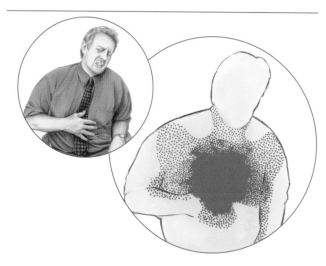

FIGURE 10. Typical locations of pain caused by a heart attack.

or that comes and goes. The uncomfortable feeling may feel like pressure, squeezing, fullness, or pain. *If someone has an uncomfortable feeling in the chest, think heart attack!* (Figure 10)

- **An uncomfortable feeling in other areas of the upper body,** such as one or both arms, the jaw, back, neck, or stomach.

- **Shortness of breath.**

- **Other signs,** such as a cold sweat, nausea, or lightheadedness.

Critical Facts

If You Suspect a Heart Attack, Phone the Emergency Response Number

A person having a heart attack is usually awake and can talk but may have an uncomfortable feeling, such as pain or pressure, in the chest. The first 60 minutes of a heart attack are the most important because that is when the victim is likely to get worse. If you think that someone may be having a heart attack, phone your company's emergency response number (or 911) right away. Minutes count!

Critical Facts

Signs of Heart Attack in Women, the Elderly, and People With Diabetes

Signs of a heart attack are often less clear in women, the elderly, and people with diabetes. These people may describe the uncomfortable feeling in the chest as an ache, heartburn, or indigestion, or the uncomfortable feeling may be in the back, jaw, neck, or shoulder.

Actions for Chest Pain and Heart Attack

Many people with an uncomfortable feeling in the chest will not admit that it may be caused by a heart attack. People often say, "I'm too healthy," "I don't want to bother the doctor," "I don't want to frighten my wife," or "I'll feel ridiculous if it isn't a heart attack." If the victim does not act, **you**—the rescuer—must act.

1. Have the victim sit quietly.

2. Phone or have someone phone your company's emergency response number (or 911).

3. Ask someone to get the AED (if your company has one) and the First Aid Kit.

4. Be ready to do CPR and use the AED if the victim becomes unresponsive.

FYI...

Sudden Cardiac Arrest

Heart disease is the single biggest cause of death in the United States. Each year about 250,000 of these deaths occur when the heart suddenly stops beating **(sudden cardiac arrest).** Sudden cardiac arrest after a heart attack is most likely during the *first hour* after the signs of a heart attack begin. So it is important that you phone the emergency response number as soon as you suspect that someone is having a heart attack. A person having a heart attack is less likely to die if you start the American Heart Association Chain of Survival immediately by phoning for help and being prepared to start CPR and use an AED.

Case Example (continued)

At the beginning of this chapter about Heart Attacks, you read this Case Example:

A middle-aged co-worker complains of an uncomfortable feeling of pressure in his chest, which he has had for the last 15 minutes. You introduce yourself and ask if you may help. You notice that he is short of breath.

You read this question: Would you know what to do?

Now you know what to do.

You ask your co-worker to sit quietly while you phone your company's emergency response number. He says, "Don't bother anyone. It's probably just something I ate." You ignore him and continue to phone.

C h a p t e r *Farthing* *Fainting*

Case Example

A co-worker is squatting in front of the bottom shelf, looking for equipment. He stands up suddenly, grabs some boxes, and then falls to the ground. As you walk toward him, you see that his eyes are closed and he is not moving. By the time you get to him, he is moving and says, "I'm OK."

Would you know what to do?

What You Will Learn

By the end of this chapter you should be able to

- Describe what fainting is
- Describe the first aid actions for fainting

Signs of Fainting

Fainting is a short period of unresponsiveness. Before becoming unresponsive the victim feels dizzy. The unresponsiveness lasts less than a minute, and then the victim seems fine.

Fainting often occurs when the victim

- Stands without moving for a long time, especially if it is hot
- Suddenly stands after squatting or bending down
- Receives bad news

Actions for Fainting

If a person is dizzy but is still responsive:

1. Make sure the area is safe.
2. Help the victim lie flat on the floor.

If a person faints and then becomes responsive:

1. Ask the victim to lie flat on the floor until all dizziness goes away.
2. If the victim remains dizzy, raise the victim's legs about 12 inches and keep them elevated until the victim is no longer dizzy.
3. Look for injuries caused by the victim's fall.
4. Once the victim is no longer dizzy, help the victim to sit up very slowly and briefly remain sitting before slowly getting up.

Case Example (continued)

At the beginning of this chapter about Fainting, you read the following Case Example:

A co-worker is squatting in front of the bottom shelf, looking for equipment. He stands up suddenly, grabs some boxes and then slumps to the ground. As you walk toward him, you see that his eyes are closed and he is not moving. By the time you get to him, he is moving and says, "I'm OK."

You read this question: Would you know what to do?

Now you know what to do.

You introduce yourself and ask if you may help. You ask the victim to continue to lie down. After a few minutes, you ask the victim if he is dizzy. When he tells you that he is not dizzy, you help him sit up slowly and then you help him to stand. After the victim sits up slowly and then stands up with your help, he says that he is fine and thanks you. You ask him to lie down again if he feels dizzy.

Chapter Diabetes and Low Blood Sugar

Case Example

Your team has worked without a lunch break and it is late afternoon. You notice that one of your team members has become very angry during the meeting. She is pale and sweating, although the room is not especially warm. She then looks tired and gets quieter. You ask if you may help. She tells you that she feels very sleepy. She says she is a diabetic and probably should have eaten by now.

Would you know what to do?

What You Will Learn

By the end of this chapter you should be able to

- Describe the signs of low blood sugar in a diabetic
- Describe the first aid actions for low blood sugar in a diabetic

FYI...

Insulin and Low Blood Sugar

Insulin helps turn sugar into energy. Since people with diabetes do not make enough insulin, they give themselves insulin injections. If a person with diabetes doesn't eat enough sugar for the amount of insulin injected, the sugar level in the blood drops. Low blood sugar causes the victim's behavior to change.

Low Blood Sugar

Low blood sugar can occur if a person with diabetes

- Has not eaten

- Has not eaten enough food for the level of activity (such as exercise)
- Has injected too much insulin

Signs of Low Blood Sugar

Signs of low blood sugar can appear quickly and may include

- A change in behavior, such as confusion or irritability
- Sleepiness or even unresponsiveness
- Hunger, thirst, or weakness
- Sweating, pale skin color
- A seizure (see Chapter 6 in this section)

Actions for Low Blood Sugar

If the victim can swallow:

1. Give the victim something containing sugar to eat or drink. This can be fruit juice, a packet of sugar, or a soda *(do not use sugar-free or diet soda or sugar substitutes because these do not contain sugar)*.

2. Have the victim sit quietly or lie down.

3. Phone or have someone phone your company's emergency response number (or 911) if the victim does not feel better within a few minutes after eating or drinking something containing sugar.

If the victim is unresponsive:

1. Phone or have someone phone your company's emergency response number (or 911).

2. Do not give the victim anything to eat or drink.

3. Do CPR as needed.

Case Example (continued)

At the beginning of this chapter about Diabetes and Low Blood Sugar, you read the following Case Example:

Your team has worked without a lunch break and it is late afternoon. You notice that one of your team members has become very angry during the meeting. You also notice that she is pale and sweating, although the room is not especially warm. She then looks tired and gets quieter. You ask if you may help. She tells you that she feels very sleepy. She says she is a diabetic and probably should have eaten by now.

You read this question: Would you know what to do?

Now you know what to do.

You look in the refrigerator in the lounge area for a drink that contains sugar. You do not pick a diet soda. You find some orange juice and bring it to her. She drinks it and soon feels much better. She thanks you for your help.

Chapter **5** *Stroke*

Case Example

Your supervisor is talking to you. Suddenly he stops speaking, and then his right arm falls to his side. When he tries to speak, you notice that one side of his mouth is lower than the other side. After a few seconds he slumps to the ground.

Would you know what to do?

What You Will Learn

By the end of this chapter you should be able to

- List 3 signs of stroke

- Describe the first aid actions for stroke

Strokes occur when blood flow to a part of the brain is suddenly blocked. This can happen if a blood vessel in the brain is blocked or bursts. The signs of a stroke are usually very sudden.

It is important to recognize the signs of a stroke because new treatments are now available. These treatments can decrease brain damage, but they must be given in the first hours after the first signs of stroke appear.

Signs of Stroke

The 3 most common signs of stroke are

- Sudden facial droop or weakness on one side of the face

- Sudden weakness on one side of the body (one arm or leg)

- Sudden trouble speaking or understanding

Other signs may include

- Sudden numbness on one side of the body

- Sudden trouble seeing in one or both eyes

- Sudden severe headache ("the worst headache of my life")

- Sudden confusion, dizziness, and loss of balance

Actions for Stroke

1. Make sure the area is safe so that the victim does not get hurt.

2. Phone or ask someone to phone your company's emergency response number (or 911) and get the First Aid Kit.

3. If the victim is unresponsive, do CPR as needed.

Case Example (continued)

At the beginning of this chapter, you read the following Case Example:

Your supervisor is talking to you. Suddenly he stops speaking, and then his right arm falls to his side. When he tries to speak, you notice that one side of his mouth is lower than the other side. After a few seconds he slumps to the ground.

You read this question: Would you know what to do?

Now you know what to do.

You ask if you may help. He is responsive and is breathing normally, but he can't speak and is unable to move his right arm, hand, or leg. He has no signs of injury. Since no one else is present, you leave to phone your company's emergency response number and get the First Aid Kit. When you return, you continue to check his breathing until EMS rescuers arrive.

C h a p t e r *Seizure*

Case Example

You are at work and hear a cry for help. You grab your First Aid Kit and run to see what the problem is. You find a co-worker on the ground surrounded by people. The man's body, arms, and legs are jerking.

Would you know what to do?

What You Will Learn

By the end of this chapter you should be able to

- List 4 causes of a seizure

- Describe how someone may move or act if he/she is having a seizure

- Describe how you would protect someone having a seizure

- List first aid actions for a person having a seizure

A medical condition called epilepsy often causes seizures. But *not all* seizures are due to epilepsy. Seizures can also be caused by

- Head injury

- Low blood sugar

- Heat-related injury

- Poison injury

Signs of a Seizure

During a seizure the victim loses muscle control and may become unresponsive. The victim usually has jerking movements of the arms and legs and sometimes of other parts of the body.

Actions for a Seizure

Most seizures stop within a few minutes. During a seizure you should

1. Protect the victim from injury by

   a. Moving furniture or other objects out of the victim's way

   b. Placing a pad or towel under the victim's head

2. Phone or have someone phone your company's emergency response number (or 911).

After a seizure it is not unusual for the victim to be confused for a few minutes. Stay with the victim until he/she becomes fully awake.

DO NOT

When giving first aid to a victim having a seizure:

- **DO NOT** hold the victim down

- **DO NOT** put anything in the victim's mouth

Case Example (continued)

At the beginning of this chapter you read the following Case Example:

You are at work and hear a cry for help. You grab your First Aid Kit and run to see what the problem is. You find a co-worker on the ground surrounded by people. The man's body, arms, and legs are jerking.

You read this question: Would you know what to do?

Now you know what to do.

You make sure that the area is safe for the victim. You ask everyone to step back, and you put a jacket under the victim's head. Within a few minutes the jerking movements stop. You check the victim's breathing. He is breathing normally. When you ask if he can hear you, he opens his eyes and nods. At first he is confused, but then he begins to act normal.

Review Questions

1. **While eating in the cafeteria, you see someone suddenly grab his throat. He cannot cough. When you ask if he can speak, he shakes his head "no." What should you do next?**

    a. Tell him you will help and give abdominal thrusts (the Heimlich maneuver)

    b. Perform a head tilt–chin lift to open the airway

    c. Give several rescue breaths

    d. Encourage him to continue to try to cough

2. **At the annual office party a co-worker eats an egg roll. Within minutes she starts to have swelling of the face and difficulty breathing. Which of the following rescue actions SHOULD NOT be done at this time?**

    a. Open her airway and give mouth-to-mouth rescue breaths

    b. Ask her if she is allergic to anything

    c. Ask her if she has an emergency epinephrine kit

    d. Phone your company's emergency response number

3. **Your friend, who is known to have seizures, begins to have a seizure. Which of the following should be your next step?**

    a. Hold him down

    b. Place your fingers in his mouth to keep him from biting his tongue

    c. Open his airway with a head tilt–chin lift

    d. Protect the victim from injury and wait for the seizure to stop

4. **Your co-worker suddenly stops working, becomes pale and sweaty, and complains of chest pressure. Which of the following is a warning sign that he may be having a heart attack and that you should immediately phone your company's emergency response number?**

    a. Sharp, stabbing chest pain that disappears in a few seconds

    b. An uncomfortable squeezing feeling in the chest or pressure in the chest that lasts for more than 5 minutes

    c. His chest pressure goes away after he takes a pill prescribed by his doctor for chest pain

    d. A lot of belching and pain in the abdomen

5. **You are talking with your supervisor when you notice that she is suddenly slurring her words. You think she may be having a stroke. Which of the following is another common sign of stroke?**

    a. Sudden development of facial droop

    b. Sudden development of sweating and crushing chest pain that lasts more than 5 minutes

    c. No breathing or signs of circulation

    d. Sudden trouble breathing

6. **Your co-worker has diabetes and asks for your help. She says that she skipped lunch. She is sweaty, pale, and confused.**

    a. Give her some soda or juice to drink

    b. Ask her to lie quietly and rest

    c. Get the First Aid Kit and AED

    d. Help her to give herself an epinephrine injection

How did you do?

1. **The correct answer is a.** Abdominal thrusts (the Heimlich maneuver) are the treatment for choking in a victim who cannot breathe or speak.

   Answer **b** is incorrect because you open the airway with a head tilt–chin lift if the victim becomes unresponsive.

   Answer **c** is incorrect because rescue breaths are not recommended for relieving choking.

   Answer **d** is incorrect because a victim whose airway is completely blocked cannot speak and cannot cough.

2. **The correct answer is a. Note that this question asked what you SHOULD NOT do.** The victim is showing signs of a bad allergic reaction (swelling of the face and difficulty breathing). You SHOULD NOT open the victim's airway and give mouth-to-mouth rescue breaths because the victim is responsive and breathing, and that may make it harder for the victim to breathe.

   Answers **b** and **c** are incorrect because you DO want to know whether the victim has allergies and if she has an epinephrine pen with her.

   Answer **d** is incorrect because when a victim shows signs of a bad allergic reaction, you DO want to call your company's emergency response number.

3. **The correct answer is d.** When someone is having a seizure, you need to protect the victim and wait for the seizure to stop.

   Answers **a** and **b** are incorrect because you should never hold a seizure victim down or place anything in the victim's mouth.

   Answer **c** is incorrect. You open the airway if a victim is unresponsive.

4. **The correct answer is b.** One sign of a heart attack is an uncomfortable squeezing feeling in the chest or pressure in the chest that lasts for more than 5 minutes.

   Answer **a** is incorrect because sharp chest pain that disappears in a few seconds is usually not a sign of a heart attack.

   Answer **c** is incorrect because the signs of a heart attack do not disappear when the victim takes medicine.

   Answer **d** is incorrect because a lot of belching with abdominal pain is not a sign of a heart attack.

5. **The correct answer is a.** The sudden development of facial droop is a common sign of stroke.

   Answer **b** is incorrect because sweating and crushing chest pain are signs of a heart attack rather than stroke.

   Answers **c** and **d** are incorrect because stroke victims usually continue breathing and have signs of circulation.

6. **The correct answer is a.** The correct first aid action for signs of low blood sugar in a victim with diabetes is to give the victim something that contains sugar, such as juice or soda (not diet soda).

   Answer **b** is incorrect because rest is not a first aid action for low blood sugar. A person with diabetes and low blood sugar will get worse unless he/she eats or drinks some sugar.

   Answer **c** is incorrect because the victim is responsive and therefore does not need an AED, and there is nothing in the First Aid Kit that will help her. It also wastes time.

   Answer **d** is incorrect because epinephrine is not a first aid action for low blood sugar.

Injury Emergencies

Chapter ❶ Bleeding You Can See

Case Example

A co-worker is hit by a car in front of your workplace. You make sure that your company's emergency response number has been called. You get your First Aid Kit and run to help. You check the scene to make sure it is safe. You ask a bystander to stop traffic. The victim is responsive and complains of pain in her arm and stomach area.

Would you know what to do?

What You Will Learn

By the end of this chapter you should be able to

- Tell why it is important to stop bleeding quickly

- List the first aid actions for bleeding that you can see

- Show how to

  — Put a pressure dressing on a bleeding area

  — Lift a bleeding arm or leg above the level of the heart

  — Apply a bandage over a dressing

- Tell how to stop bleeding from the nose and the mouth

- Describe the first aid for an amputated part of the body

Actions for Bleeding You Can See

Bleeding is one of the most frightening emergencies. Many cuts are small and the bleeding can be easily stopped, but when a large blood vessel is cut or torn, the victim can lose a large amount of blood within minutes. That's why you have to act fast.

Remember:

- Remain calm.

- You can stop most bleeding with pressure.

- Bleeding often looks a lot worse than it is.

Take the following actions to stop bleeding that you can see:

1. Make sure that the area is safe for you and the victim.

2. Send someone to get the First Aid Kit.

3. Wear personal protective equipment.

4. If the victim is able, ask the victim to put pressure over the wound with a large clean dressing while you put on gloves and eye shield.

5. *You should be able to stop most bleeding with pressure alone.* Put pressure on the dressing

over the bleeding area with the flat part of your fingers or the palm of your hand (Figure 1A-C). A small amount of pressure is all that you need to control bleeding from a scrape. You have to press harder to stop severe bleeding. If the bleeding does not stop, add a second dressing and press harder. Do not take a dressing off once it is in place. If you remove the first dressing, it might pull off some blood clots and cause the wound to bleed more. If a dressing becomes soaked with blood, add more dressings and press harder (Figure 2).

6. If the bleeding is from a wound on an arm or leg, raise the arm or leg so that it is higher than the chest while you continue to put pressure on the wound (Figure 3). Do not raise the arm or leg if movement causes the victim pain.

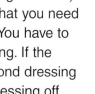
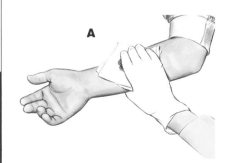
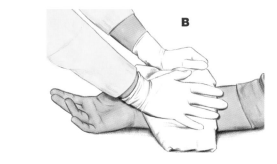
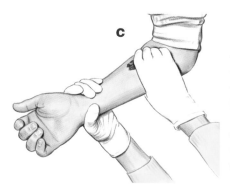

FIGURE 1.
A dressing can be a gauze pad (A) or any other clean piece of cloth (B). If you do not have a dressing, you may even use your gloved hand (C).

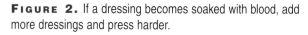
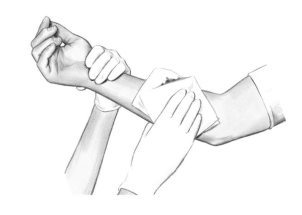

FIGURE 2. If a dressing becomes soaked with blood, add more dressings and press harder.

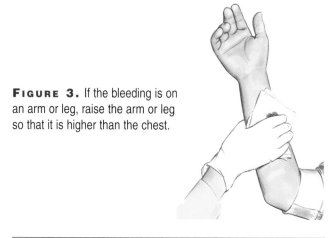

FIGURE 3. If the bleeding is on an arm or leg, raise the arm or leg so that it is higher than the chest.

7. Check for signs of shock and give first aid as needed (see Chapter 2 in this section).

8. Phone or ask someone to phone your company's emergency response number (or 911) if

- There is a lot of bleeding

- You cannot stop the bleeding

- You are not sure what to do

Case Example (continued)

At the beginning of this chapter about Bleeding That You Can See, you read the following Case Example:

A co-worker is hit by a car in front of your workplace. You make sure that your company's emergency response number has been called. You get your First Aid Kit and run to help. You check the scene to make sure it is safe. You ask a bystander to stop traffic. The victim is responsive and complains of pain in her arm and stomach area.

You read this question: Would you know what to do?

Now you know what to do.

You identify yourself and ask for permission to help. You check the victim and note that she is alert, breathing normally, and bleeding from her right arm. You ask the victim to put pressure on the bleeding area of her arm while you put on gloves and an eye shield. You quickly put pressure on the bleeding area with your gloved hand. Then you apply strong pressure over a sterile dressing. You look for signs of shock.

Special Areas of Bleeding That You Can See

Bleeding From the Nose

Nosebleeds are common. It can be hard to know how much bleeding there is because the victim often swallows some of the blood. If the victim vomits, blood can block the windpipe and cause breathing problems.

Actions for Nosebleeds

1. Make sure the area is safe for you and the victim. Send someone to get the First Aid Kit.

2. Put on personal protective equipment.

3. Press both sides of the victim's nostrils while the victim sits and leans *forward* (Figure 4).

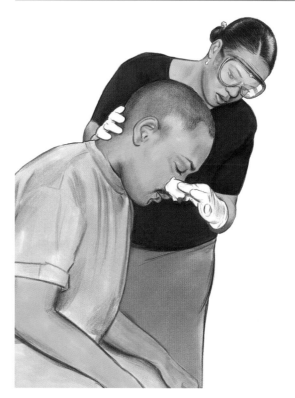

FIGURE 4. To stop a nosebleed, press both sides of the victim's nostrils while the victim sits and leans forward.

4. Place constant pressure on both sides of the nostrils for a few minutes.

5. If bleeding continues, press harder and hold pressure.

6. Phone or ask someone to phone your company's emergency response number (or 911) if

   - You can't stop the bleeding in about 15 minutes

   - The victim has trouble breathing

Bleeding From the Mouth

Like other bleeding you can see, bleeding from the mouth can usually be stopped with pressure. But bleeding from the mouth can be serious if blood or broken teeth block the airway and cause breathing problems or if you can't reach the bleeding area.

Actions for Bleeding From the Mouth

1. Make sure that the area is safe for you and the victim. Send someone to get the First Aid Kit.

2. Put on personal protective equipment.

3. If the bleeding is from the tongue, lip, or cheek or another area you can easily reach, press the bleeding area with a sterile gauze or clean cloth (Figure 5).

4. If bleeding is deep in the mouth and you can't reach it easily, place the victim on his/her side.

5. Look for signs of shock (see Chapter 2 in this section).

6. Check the victim's airway and breathing. Be ready to start CPR if needed.

7. Phone or ask someone to phone your company's emergency response number (or 911) if

   - You can't stop the bleeding
   - The victim has trouble breathing

Amputations

If a part of the body, such as a finger, toe, hand, or foot is cut off (amputated), you should save the body part because doctors may be able to re-attach it. You can preserve a detached body part at room temperature, but it will be in a better condition to be reattached if you keep it cool.

Actions for Amputation

1. Make sure that the area is safe for you and the victim.

2. Phone or ask someone to phone your company's emergency response number (or 911) and get the First Aid Kit.

3. Put on personal protective equipment.

4. Stop the bleeding from the stump with direct pressure.

5. Watch for signs of shock and give first aid as needed (see Chapter 2 in this section).

6. If you can find the amputated part, rinse it with sterile or clean water (Figure 6A). Then cover or wrap it with a clean dressing. If it will fit, place it in a watertight plastic bag (Figure 6B). Place that bag in another container with ice or ice and water, label it with the victim's name, date, and time (Figure 6C), and make sure it is sent to the hospital with the victim. *Never place the amputated body part directly on ice because the cold may damage it.*

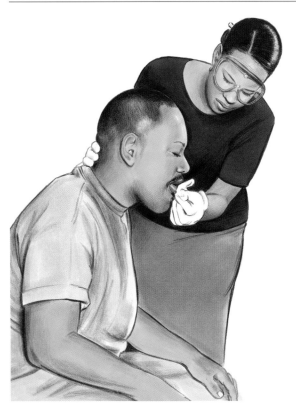

FIGURE 5. If the bleeding is from the tongue, lip, or cheek, press the bleeding area with a sterile gauze or clean cloth.

FIGURE 6. A, If you can find the amputated part, rinse it with sterile or clean water. Then cover or wrap it with a clean dressing. **B,** If it will fit, place it in a watertight plastic bag. **C,** Place that bag in another container with ice or ice and water, label it with the victim's name, date, and time, and make sure it is sent to the hospital with the victim.

A

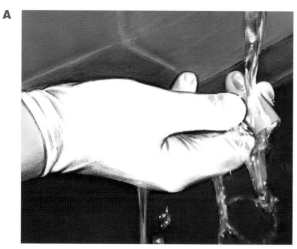

B

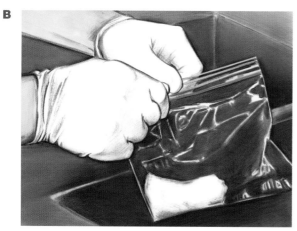

C

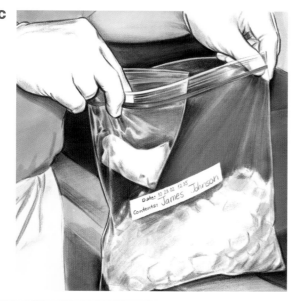

Case Example

You are giving first aid to a victim of a car crash. The victim complains of pain in her abdomen. You notice that she is becoming restless. Her skin is pale, cool, and moist. She says she is cold and complains of being sick to her stomach.

Would you know what to do?

What You Will Learn

By the end of this chapter you should be able to

- Tell what shock is
- List the signs of shock
- List the first aid actions for shock
- Tell when you should suspect bleeding inside the body

Shock

Shock develops when there is not enough blood flowing to the cells of the body. In adults shock is most often present if

- The victim loses a lot of blood that you can see or that you can't see
- The victim has a severe heart attack
- The victim has a bad allergic reaction

Signs of Shock

A victim in shock may

- Feel cold and shiver
- Feel weak, faint, or dizzy
- Be restless, agitated, or confused
- Vomit
- Feel thirsty

FYI...

Understanding the Signs of Shock

When a victim loses a lot of blood or when the victim's blood does not circulate properly, there is not enough blood delivered to the cells of the body. We call this condition "shock." In many forms of shock some blood is pumped to the most important organs of the body— the brain and heart—and less blood is pumped to the skin and muscles. As a result, the victim's skin becomes cool, pale, and sweaty. The victim may vomit or feel thirsty. If the victim loses a lot of blood quickly, there may not even be enough blood for the heart and brain, and the victim may feel afraid, restless, weak, faint, or dizzy.

Actions for Shock

If a victim has signs of shock, you should perform the following first aid actions:

1. Be sure the area is safe for you and the victim.

2. Phone or ask someone to phone your company's emergency response number (or 911) and get the First Aid Kit.

3. Help the victim lie on his/her back.

4. If there is no leg injury or pain, raise the victim's legs about 12 inches (Figure 7).

5. Use pressure to stop bleeding that you can see.

6. Cover the victim with a blanket to keep the victim warm (you can use the Mylar blanket if there is one in the First Aid Kit).

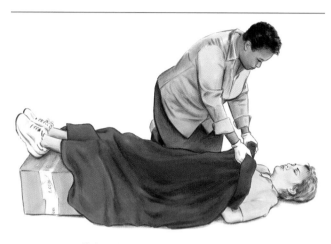

FIGURE 7. If there is no leg injury or pain, raise the victim's legs about 12 inches. Cover the victim with a blanket to keep the victim warm.

Case Example (continued)

At the beginning of this chapter on Shock, you read the following Case Example:

You are giving first aid to a victim of a car crash. The victim complains of pain in her abdomen. You notice that she is becoming restless. Her skin is pale, cool, and moist. She says she is cold and complains of being sick to her stomach.

You read this question: Would you know what to do?

Now you know what to do.

You make sure that the area is safe for you and the victim. You ask someone to direct traffic away from the area. You ask another person to phone your company's emergency response number (or 911) and get the First Aid Kit. You decide that the victim has signs of shock. She is already lying down on her back. She has no signs of leg injury or hip pain. You raise her legs about 12 inches by putting a box under them. You cover her with a blanket from the First Aid Kit. You keep looking to make sure she remains responsive. EMS rescuers arrive and treat her.

Bleeding You Can't See

A forceful blow to the chest or abdomen can injure the heart, lungs, liver, and other organs. It can cause a lot of bleeding inside the body. You may not see signs of this bleeding on the outside of the body at all, or you may see a bruise of the skin over the injured part of the body. An injury inside of the body may be minor or very severe.

When to Suspect Bleeding You Can't See

Suspect bleeding inside the body, "Bleeding You Can't See," if a victim has

- An injury from a car crash, a blast, a pedestrian injury, or a fall from a height
- A knife or gunshot wound

You should also suspect bleeding inside the body if

- The victim has an injury to the abdomen or chest
- The victim has bruises on the abdomen or chest (for example, seat belt marks or fist marks)
- The victim has pain in the chest or abdomen after an injury
- The victim coughs up or vomits blood after an injury
- The victim has signs of shock without bleeding that you can see

Actions for Bleeding You Can't See

1. Make sure that the area is safe for you and the victim.
2. Phone or ask someone to phone your company's emergency response number (or 911) and get the First Aid Kit.
3. Keep the victim still and lying down.
4. Check for signs of shock and give first aid as needed.
5. If the victim becomes unresponsive, send someone to get the AED and begin CPR.

Case Example (continued)

In Case Examples earlier in Chapter 1 and this chapter, you read about a co-worker struck by a car:

A co-worker is hit by a car in front of your workplace. You make sure that your company's emergency response number (or 911) has been called. You get your First Aid Kit and run to help. You check the scene to make sure it is safe. You ask a bystander to stop traffic.

The victim is responsive and complains of pain in her arm and stomach area. You stop the bleeding from the victim's arm and watch for signs of shock. The victim continues to complain of pain in the stomach area and become restless. Her skin is pale, cool, and moist. She is cold and sick to her stomach. You give her first aid for shock. She continues to have pain in her stomach area.

You read the question: Would you know what to do?

Now you know what to do.

You think that the victim probably has bleeding inside the abdomen. You keep looking to make sure she remains responsive. You stay with her until EMS rescuers arrive.

Case Example

A worker was unloading a truck when he was hit on the head by a forklift. When you arrive he is lying on the ground. A crowd has gathered. You quickly look around. You note that the area is safe for you and the victim. The forklift is not in the way, and there is no moving traffic. You ask someone to phone your company's emergency response number (or 911) and get the First Aid Kit. You ask another person to direct traffic away from the area. You kneel by the victim's side and gently shake him and shout. He is unresponsive.

Would you know what to do?

What You Will Learn

By the end of this chapter you should be able to

- List 6 types of injuries that are likely to result in a head injury
- List 6 signs of head injury
- List 3 types of injuries that might cause a spine injury
- Show how to open the airway of an unresponsive victim with a head or neck injury
- List first aid actions for a victim with a head and possible spinal cord injury

Head Injury

The brain is very likely to be injured whenever a victim has a blow to the head. You should suspect that the victim has a head injury if

- The victim fell from a height
- The victim was injured by a strong blow to the head
- The victim was injured while diving
- The victim was electrocuted
- The victim was involved in a high impact car crash
- The victim's helmet is broken

Signs of Head Injury

You should suspect that a victim has had a head injury if after an injury the victim

- Is unresponsive, sleepy, or confused
- Vomits
- Complains of a headache
- Has difficulty seeing
- Has difficulty moving any part of the body
- Has a seizure

Spine Injury

The bones of the spine protect the spinal cord. The spinal cord carries messages between the brain and the body. If these bones are broken, the spinal cord may be injured. The victim may not be able to move his/her legs or arms and may lose feeling in parts of the body. Some people call this a "broken back." You may cause further injury to the spinal cord if you bend, twist, or turn the victim's head or neck. When you give first aid to a victim with a possible spine injury, you must not bend, twist, or turn the head or neck.

When to Suspect Spine Injury

You should suspect that the spine bones are broken if a victim

- Has an injury to the upper part of the body, especially the head or chest
- Was injured by a falling object, a forceful blow to the head or chest, a motor vehicle crash, or a fall from a height

- Was injured while under the influence of drugs or alcohol

Actions for Head and Spine Injury

When giving first aid to a victim with a possible head injury:

1. Make sure that the area is safe for you and the victim.

2. Phone or ask someone to phone your company's emergency response number (or 911) and get the First Aid Kit.

3. Do not allow the victim's head or neck to move in any direction:

- Hold the head and neck so that the head and neck do not move, bend, or twist (Figure 8).

- Do not move the victim unless the victim is in danger or unless you need to do so to check breathing or provide CPR or if the victim is vomiting.

- If you must turn the victim, be sure to roll the victim while you support the victim's head, neck, and trunk so that the head and neck are kept in line and do not twist, bend, or turn in any direction. This requires two rescuers (Figure 9).

- If the victim is unresponsive, open the airway with a **_jaw thrust._** The jaw thrust opens the airway without moving the head and neck. Place your fingers on the angles of the jaw, and lift the jaw forward. This moves the tongue away from the back of the throat and opens the airway (Figure 10). After opening the airway, check for breathing and continue CPR as needed.

- If the victim is responsive and vomiting, roll him/her onto the side while holding the head and neck so that the head and neck do not bend or twist (Figure 9).

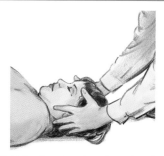

FIGURE 8. Hold the head and neck so that the head and neck do not move, bend, or twist.

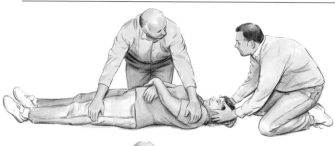

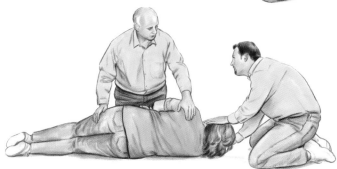

FIGURE 9. If you must turn the victim, be sure to roll the victim while you support the victim's head, neck, and trunk so that the head and neck are kept in line and do not twist, bend, or turn in any direction.

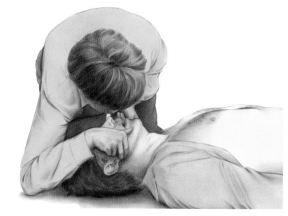

FIGURE 10. Open the airway with a jaw thrust. The jaw thrust opens the airway without moving the head and neck. Place your fingers on the angles of the jaw, and lift the jaw to move the jaw forward. This moves the tongue away from the back of the throat and opens the airway.

Case Example (continued)

At the beginning of this chapter on Head and Spine Injury, you read the following Case Example:

A worker was unloading a truck when he was hit on the head by a forklift. When you arrive he is lying on the ground. A crowd has gathered. You quickly look around. You note that the area is safe for you and the victim. The forklift is not in the way, and there is no moving traffic. You ask someone to phone your company's emergency response number (or 911) and get the First Aid Kit. You ask another person to direct traffic away from the area. You kneel by the victim's side and gently shake him and shout. He is not responsive.

You read this question: Would you know what to do?

Now you know what to do.

You open the victim's airway with a jaw thrust and check his breathing. He is breathing normally. When EMS rescuers arrive, they begin their care of the victim, and you tell them what happened.

Case Example

While playing basketball, a co-worker falls and twists her ankle. When you arrive, she is sitting on the floor in pain. Her ankle is beginning to swell and is a bluish color.

Would you know what to do?

What You Will Learn

By the end of this chapter you should be able to

- List the first aid actions for injuries to the joints and muscles

- Show how to apply ice to an injured joint

Bone, Joint, and Muscle Injuries

Injuries to bones, joints, and muscles are common in our active society. The injuries may include joint injuries, broken bones, and bruises (black-and-blue spots). Without an x-ray, it may be impossible to tell whether a bone is broken, and the information is not important when giving first aid.

Actions for Injuries to Bones, Joints, or Muscles

When giving first aid for a bone, joint, or muscle injury:

1. Make sure that the area is safe for you and the victim and get the First Aid Kit.

2. Cover an open wound with a clean dressing.

3. Check for signs of shock and give first aid as needed.

4. Don't try to straighten any injured part that is bent (such as an arm, a leg, or a finger).

5. Put a plastic bag filled with ice on the injured area with a towel between the ice bag and the skin (Figure 11). Every 20 minutes take off the ice bag for about 5 minutes. You may use a chemical cold pack, but it is not as cold and does not work as well as ice.

6. Wrap an elastic bandage around an injured joint.

7. Phone or ask someone to phone your company's emergency response number (or 911) if

   - There is a large open wound

   - The injured part is abnormally bent

   - You're not sure what to do

8. The victim should not walk on an injured foot or leg until checked by a healthcare provider.

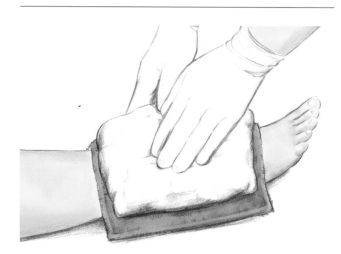

FIGURE 11. Put a plastic bag filled with ice on the injured area with a towel between the ice bag and the skin.

Joint Sprains

Joint sprains result from a twisting injury. The twisting injury causes tears in muscles and other structures around the joint. The tears cause pain, swelling, and a blue color over the joint. Ice and rest decrease the amount of joint pain and swelling and help the joint to heal faster.

Case Example (continued)

At the beginning of this chapter about Injuries to Bones, Joints, or Muscles, you read this Case Example:

While playing basketball, a co-worker falls and twists her ankle. When you arrive, she is sitting on the floor in pain. Her ankle is beginning to swell and is a bluish color.

You read this question: Would you know what to do?

Now you know what to do.

You introduce yourself and ask if you may help. You ask the victim to continue sitting on the floor. You ask someone to get the First Aid Kit. You ask a second person to get you some ice in a plastic bag. You put a towel on the ankle and put the ice bag on the towel. You hold the ice bag on the joint and take it off every 20 minutes. You then wrap an elastic bandage around the ankle. You ask the victim to lean on a colleague and not walk on the foot until she is checked by a healthcare provider.

Injury Emergencies

Causes of Burns

Burns are injuries that can be caused by contact with heat, electricity, and chemicals (see Poison Emergencies).

Case Example

A co-worker screams when she spills very hot coffee over her right hand and arm.

Would you know what to do?

What You Will Learn

By the end of this chapter you should be able to

- List the first aid actions for burns caused by heat
- List the dangers for the rescuer when giving first aid for a victim of high-voltage electrocution
- List the first aid actions for a victim of electrocution

Burns Caused by Heat

Heat burns can be caused by contact with fire, a hot surface, a hot liquid, or steam.

Actions for Burns Caused by Heat

1. Make sure that the area is safe for you and the victim, and get the First Aid Kit.

2. If the victim's clothing is on fire, have the victim "stop, drop, and roll." This smothers the flames. Running fans the flames. Cover the victim with a blanket and soak with water. Once the fire is out, remove burned clothing and jewelry from the burned area if they are not stuck to the skin.

3. If the victim is unresponsive, begin CPR as needed.

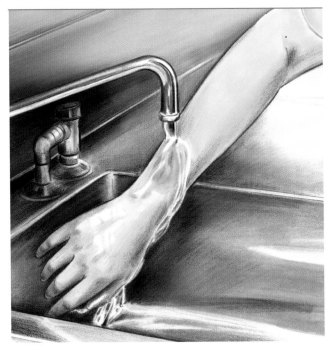

FIGURE 12. If possible, hold the burned area under cold tap water for about 15 to 30 minutes.

4. If the burn area is small, cool it immediately with cold, but not ice cold, water. If possible, hold the burned area under cold tap water for about 15 to 30 minutes (Figure 12).

5. You may cover the burn with a dry, non-sticking sterile or clean dressing.

6. Phone or ask someone to phone your company's emergency response number (or 911) if

   - There is a fire
   - A victim has a large burn
   - You are not sure what to do

Case Example (continued)

At the start of this chapter on Burns, you read this Case Example:

A co-worker screams when she spills very hot coffee over her right hand and arm.

You read this question: Would you know what to do?

Now you know what to do.

You introduce yourself and ask if you may help. You send someone to get the First Aid Kit. You roll up the co-worker's sleeve and see a red burned area. You ask the co-worker to put her hand and arm under cold tap water and cool the burn for 15 to 30 minutes. You then cover the burn with a clean, dry dressing.

Electrocution and Electrical Injury

Electricity occurs naturally in the form of lightning or from man-made sources like an electrical current. Electricity can cause burns on the surface and injure organs inside the body. If electricity enters the body, it can cause severe damage in its path and even stop the heart. You may see marks or wounds where the electricity has entered and left the body. These marks may seem very small, but *you can't tell from the outside of the body how much damage there is inside the body!*

Actions for Electrical Injury

In giving first aid for an electrical injury:

1. Do not touch the victim as long as the victim is in contact with the power source. Electricity can travel from the source through the victim to you. It's best to turn off the main power switch (usually located near the fuse box).

   If the electrocution is caused by **high voltage,** such as a fallen power line, immediately notify the proper authorities (call 911). *Remember that if the voltage is high enough, it can travel through **everything** that touches the power line or source (even a wooden stick) and can hurt you.* **Don't enter the area around the victim.** Don't try to pull away wires or other materials until the power has been turned off.

2. Phone or ask someone to phone your company's emergency response number (or 911) and get an AED if your company has one.

3. If the victim becomes unresponsive, begin CPR and use the AED if indicated.

4. Check for signs of shock and give the proper first aid (see Chapter 2 in this section).

5. All victims with an electric injury should be checked by a healthcare provider.

Review Questions

1. **You are helping a co-worker who is bleeding a lot from a large, deep cut of his hand. You have already phoned your company's emergency response number. You have brought the First Aid Kit, and you have stopped the bleeding with pressure. Now the victim is responsive but he is irritable, sweaty, pale, and cool. Which of the following first aid actions should you do *first*?**

   a. Open the victim's airway and give rescue breaths

   b. Take the dressings off the cut and check it again

   c. Put more pressure on the wound

   d. Ask the victim to lie down, raise his feet about 12 inches, and cover him with a blanket

2. **A co-worker has cut her arm. You arrive with the First Aid Kit. Which of the following first aid actions should you perform *first*?**

   a. Phone your company's emergency response number and wait until help arrives

   b. Put pressure on the bleeding area with your bare hand over a dressing

   c. Ask the victim to put pressure over a dressing on the cut while you put on protective gloves

   d. Raise the victim's arm above the level of the heart before putting pressure on the bleeding area

3. **A co-worker has a nosebleed and asks for your help. Which of the following steps would be best for you to perform *first?***

   a. Ask the victim to lie down

   b. Ask the victim to sit up and lean forward

   c. Ask the victim to sit up and lean his head way back

   d. Ask the victim to cough

4. **A co-worker has cut off his finger. Another first aid rescuer is applying pressure to the man's hand and has stopped the bleeding. You locate the finger. Which of the following correctly describes the *best* actions that you should take with the finger?**

   a. Leave the finger where you found it because it's dirty

   b. Put the finger in a plastic bag and send it with the victim to the hospital

   c. Wash the finger, put it on a piece of ice, put it in a plastic bag, label it with the victim's name, and send it with the victim to the hospital

   d. Wash the finger, put it in a plastic bag, put the plastic bag into another bag that has ice in it, label the outside bag with the victim's name, and send it with the victim to the hospital

5. **A victim of a high-speed car crash seems OK, but she complains of pain in her abdomen. You see a black-and-blue mark on her abdomen. Which of the following should you do?**

   a. Suspect that the victim may have bleeding inside the abdomen and phone your company's emergency response number

   b. Put pressure on the black-and-blue area on the victim's abdomen to stop any bleeding

   c. Reassure the victim that she is fine

   d. Ask the victim to stand up and see if she can walk

6. A worker fell from high scaffolding and is unresponsive. He is lying on his back. A co-worker has left to phone the company's emergency response number and bring the First Aid Kit and the AED. You remain with the victim. Which of the following should you do *first*?

   a. Open his airway using a head tilt–chin lift

   b. Move his neck first to see if it causes him pain

   c. Open his airway with a jaw thrust, being careful not to move his head or neck

   d. Move him away from the scene of the injury before you do anything else

7. You are playing basketball when another player falls and twists his ankle. The ankle is beginning to swell. The player asks you to help. Which of the following first aid actions would be best?

   a. Put a towel on the ankle and keep ice over the towel for about 20 minutes

   b. Help the player walk to the nearest health-care facility

   c. Reassure the player and tell him he'll be fine

   d. Wrap a bandage around the player's ankle

8. Your co-worker spills hot liquid on her arm, burning it. She asks for your help. Which of the following first aid actions would be best?

   a. Put ice on the burn

   b. Smear butter or petroleum jelly on the burn area as soon as possible

   c. Wrap the burn area with a dressing

   d. Rinse the burn area with cold water from the faucet for 15 to 30 minutes

9. A worker gets an electric shock while working with a tool. When you arrive he is responsive and says he is fine, but he complains of a headache. You see a small bruise on his forehead. Which of the following would be the best first aid actions for you to take?

   a. Reassure him that he'll be fine

   b. Strongly urge him to seek medical attention because neither he nor you can tell what kind of injury the shock may have caused

   c. Put pressure on the bruise to stop any bleeding

   d. Send someone to get an AED

How did you do?

1. **The correct answer is d.** The victim is showing signs of shock. He has lost a large amount of blood, and he is irritable, sweaty, and cold. The correct first aid for shock is to help the victim lie down, raise the victim's feet, and cover the victim with a blanket.

   Answer **a** is incorrect because the victim is responsive and breathing, so there is no need to open the airway or give rescue breaths.

   Answer **b** is incorrect because you should not remove dressings from a bleeding area. In doing so you may pull off clots and restart the bleeding.

   Answer **c** is incorrect because the bleeding has stopped and there is no reason to put more dressings on the wound.

2. **The correct answer is c.** You should ask the victim to put pressure over the bleeding cut while you put on protective gloves.

   Answer **a** is incorrect because you should try to stop the bleeding before you phone the company's emergency response number unless the victim is in shock or unresponsive.

Answer **b** is incorrect because if you have the First Aid Kit, you should put on protective gloves when you think you might come in contact with a victim's blood or body fluids.

Answer **d** is incorrect because you don't raise the arm first. You do that if pressure and adding more dressings don't work.

3. **The correct answer is b.** When you are trying to stop a nosebleed, the victim should be sitting up and leaning *forward*.

Answers **a** and **c** are incorrect because the victim should not lie down or lean his head back.

Answer **d** is incorrect because coughing can make the bleeding worse.

4. **The correct answer is d.** If a body part has been amputated, you should wash it, put it in a plastic bag, put the plastic bag in another bag that has ice in it, label it with the victim's name, date, and time and send it with the victim to the hospital.

Answer **a** is incorrect because you should not leave the body part, no matter what its condition, even if you don't think it can be reattached. You should leave it only if getting it would put you in danger.

Answer **b** is incorrect because you should try to preserve the body part. Although the body part can be left at room temperature, it is best to keep it cold.

Answer **c** is incorrect because you should not put the part directly on ice because the cold may damage it.

5. **The correct answer is a.** This is a good example of possible bleeding you cannot see. The victim was involved in a high-speed car crash and has abdominal pain. If you think there may be bleeding inside the body, you should immediately phone your company's emergency response number.

Answer **b** is incorrect because putting pressure on the black-and-blue area of the victim's abdomen will not stop the bleeding inside the body, and it may cause further pain.

Answer **c** is incorrect because you should not simply reassure the victim.

Answer **d** is incorrect because you certainly should not ask the victim to stand and walk, which might make the bleeding worse.

6. **The correct answer is c.** Because the victim fell from a height and is unresponsive, you should consider that he may have a spine injury. For this reason you should open the airway with a jaw thrust instead of a head tilt–chin lift to avoid moving the head and neck. You should also be prepared to provide CPR and use the AED (if your company has one).

Answers **a, b,** and **d** are incorrect because you should not move the victim at all unless the victim is in danger or you need to move the victim to check breathing or start CPR. If you do move the victim, you should prevent the neck from bending or twisting. When you open the airway you should use a jaw thrust instead of a head tilt–chin lift.

7. **The correct answer is a.** You should put ice in or on a towel and place the towel on the victim's ankle.

Answers **b, c,** and **d** are incorrect because waiting to put ice on the ankle will mean that it will take longer for the ankle to heal and the victim will be in pain for a longer time.

8. **The correct answer is d.** You should immediately cool the burn with water from a faucet.

Answers **a** and **b** are incorrect because ice can damage the skin, and petroleum jelly and butter seal the heat in the burn area, so they may make it worse.

Answer **c** is incorrect because cooling causes the burn to hurt less and heal faster. Wrapping the burn without cooling is not enough to help.

9. **The correct answer is b.** You can't tell whether there is any damage inside the body. For this reason answer **a** is incorrect because you should not simply reassure the victim.

Answer **c** is incorrect because putting pressure on the bruise does nothing for an injury inside the body.

Answer **d** is incorrect because the AED is not needed since the victim is responsive and the immediate danger from electrocution is over.

Appendix
Practice Sessions

During the course you will have practice sessions and you will be asked to refer to the following.

Bleeding You Can See

During the practice session, participants work in pairs and take turns role-playing the victim and rescuer.

Victim is bleeding from the arm.

Rescuer: "I'm trained in first aid. May I help you?"

- Gives victim gauze dressing and asks victim to apply pressure over bleeding area while rescuer puts on gloves.
- Applies pressure over gauze.
- Adds more gauze and applies pressure.
- Raises bleeding area while continuing to apply pressure.
- Applies bandage over dressing to maintain pressure.

Shock

During the practice session, participants work in pairs and take turns role-playing victim and rescuer.

The **victim** is lying down and is asked by the rescuer to describe his/her signs of shock according to the following script.

Rescuer: "My name is _____ and I'm trained in first aid. May I help you? How do you feel?"

Victim: "Lousy! I'm shivering with cold. I feel like I'm going to throw up. I'm dizzy and very thirsty." The victim then checks that the rescuer performs correct actions. Do not interrupt the rescuer. Wait until the rescuer has finished and then point out if anything has been skipped or done incorrectly.

Rescuer

- Asks someone to phone the company emergency response number (or 911).
- Raises the victim's feet about 12 inches unless there is a leg injury.
- Covers the victim with a blanket.
- Tells the victim that help is on the way.

Immobilization of Head and Neck and Jaw Thrust

During the practice session, participants work in pairs and take turns role-playing victim and rescuer.

Rescuer

- Makes sure the area is safe.
- Asks bystander to phone the company emergency response number (or 911).
- Taps victim and asks, "Are you OK?" (victim is unresponsive).
- Kneels behind victim, immobilizes victim's head and neck, and opens the airway with a jaw thrust.

Victim

- Is lying down and is unresponsive.
- Checks to make sure rescuer performs all steps correctly and in proper order.

Environmental Emergencies

Chapter ❶ Bites and Stings

Case Example

You and your co-workers are working in a public park. One of them suddenly stops, bends down to look at something, and calls out, "Look at this! There's a big raccoon under this bush!" He then screams, and you realize that the raccoon has bitten his hand.

Would you know what to do?

What You Will Learn

By the end of this chapter you should be able to

■ List the first aid actions for

— A human and animal bite

— Snakebite

— An insect sting

— A spider bite

— A scorpion sting

■ Tell how to remove a tick

Animal and Human Bites

Human and animal bites can be painful. When the bite punctures the skin, the wound can bleed and become infected.

Actions for Animal and Human Bites

1. Make sure that the area is safe for you and the victim. Do not touch any part of an animal that may be rabid.

2. Phone or ask someone to phone your company's emergency response number (or 911) and get the First Aid Kit.

3. Clean the victim's wound with soap (if available) and water under pressure from a faucet.

4. Stop the bleeding by applying direct pressure.

5. Report all animal bites to the police or an animal control officer. Describe the animal, how the bite happened, and the location of the animal when last seen.

Critical Facts

Rabies

Assume that an animal has rabies if

■ The animal attacks without being provoked

■ The animal behaves in an unusual manner (for example, if a usually friendly dog attacks)

■ The animal is a skunk, raccoon, fox, bat, or other wild mammal

■ You are not sure

Case Example (continued)

At the beginning of this chapter, you read the following Case Example:

You and your co-workers are working in a public park. One of them suddenly stops, bends down to look at something, and calls out, "Look at this! There's a big raccoon under this bush!" He then screams, and you realize that the raccoon has bitten his hand.

You read the following question: Would you know what to do?

Now you know what to do.

When you run over, you see that the raccoon is slowly backing off. You think that the raccoon may be rabid because it is behaving strangely. You ask a third co-worker to phone your company's

emergency response number, and bring the First Aid Kit. You ask if you can help, and then you help your co-worker clean the wound by washing his hand with water flowing rapidly from a hose. There is slight bleeding, which you stop with pressure. EMS rescuers arrive and take your co-worker to the hospital. You immediately call the police and report that a possibly rabid raccoon is in the park.

Snakebites

Case Example

While you are working at a construction site, you are called to help a co-worker who has been bitten in the leg by a snake. The snake has disappeared.

Would you know what to do?

There are 4 poisonous snake groups in the United States:

1. Rattlesnakes, which cause most poisonous snakebites and nearly all snakebite deaths in the United States

2. Copperheads

3. Water moccasins (also called cottonmouths)

4. Coral snakes

Type of Snake

It is helpful to be able to identify the snake (Figure 1). Sometimes you can identify the snake from its bite mark or its behavior. *If you aren't sure whether a snake is poisonous, assume that it is.*

Nonpoisonous Snake

Nonpoisonous snakes leave tooth marks in the shape of a horseshoe. The bite of some nonpoisonous snakes (for example, hognose and garter snakes) can be painful and may cause swelling and redness but have no other harmful effects.

Rattlesnake, Copperhead, and Water Moccasin

These snakes (Figure 1) usually leave 2 (sometimes just 1) puncture wounds about ½ inch apart.

One fourth of the bites are "dry" bites in which no poison is injected into the victim.

Coral Snake

Coral snakes (Figure 2) are the most poisonous snakes in the United States, but they rarely bite people. They have short fangs and hang on and "chew" poison into the victim rather than strike and release.

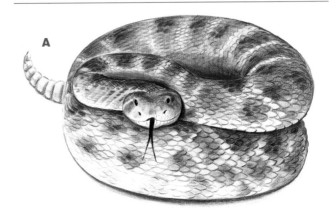
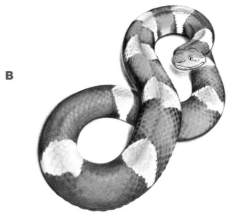
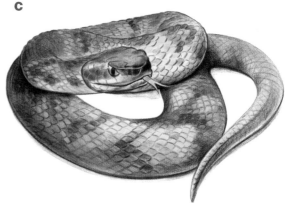

FIGURE 1. A, Rattlesnake, **B,** Copperhead and **C,** Water Moccasin.

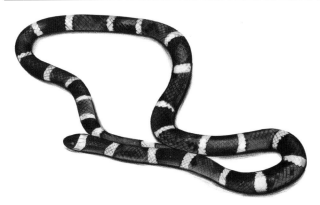

FIGURE 2. Coral Snake.

Signs of Snakebite Poisoning

If poison has been injected by snakebite, the victim will have

- Severe burning at the bite
- Swelling of the bite area within 5 minutes of the bite
- Nausea, vomiting, sweating, and weakness

Actions for Snakebite

1. Be careful around a wounded snake. Back away and go around the snake. If by accident a snake has been killed or injured, do not handle it. A snake might bite even when severely injured or close to death. If it needs to be moved, a shovel would be safest. If you don't need to move it, it is best to leave it alone.

2. Phone or ask someone to phone your company's emergency response number or 911 and bring the First Aid Kit.

3. Ask the victim to be still and calm. Tell the victim not to move the part of the body that was bitten.

4. Gently wash the victim's bite area with soap (if available) and water.

5. If the bite was caused by a coral snake, apply mild pressure by wrapping several elastic bandages over the bite and the entire arm or leg. *Do not* wrap the bite area with a dressing if any other snake caused the bite.

DO NOT

Wrong Actions for Snakebite

When you give first aid for snakebite:

- **DO NOT** apply cold or ice.
- **DO NOT** use the "cut-and-suck" procedure or any other method to remove the poison.
- **DO NOT** use local electric shock.

Critical Facts

Actions for Coral Snakebite

First aid for a coral snakebite is different than for other snakebites. As part of first aid for a coral snakebite, you should put on a pressure dressing over the bite and the whole arm or leg.

Coral snakes

- Have short fangs
- Tend to hang on and "chew" their poison into the victim rather than strike and release.

Case Example (continued)

At the beginning of this section about Snakebites, you read the following Case Example:

While you are working at a construction site, you are called to help a co-worker who has been bitten in his leg by a snake. The snake has disappeared.

You also read this question: Would you know what to do?

Now you know what to do.

You ask someone to phone your company's emergency response number or 911 and get the First Aid Kit. You make sure that the snake is not nearby and that the area is safe for you and the victim. You ask if you may help. Then you ask the victim to lie very still and not to move his leg. You put on protective gloves when the First Aid Kit arrives.

Summary of First Aid Actions for Bites

Human and Animal	Nonpoisonous Snake *or* Rattlesnake, Copperhead, and Water Moccasin	Coral Snake
1. Make sure the area is safe for you and the victim.	1. Get the victim to a safe area away from the snake. Make sure the area is safe for you and the victim.	
2. Phone your company's emergency response number or 911 and get the First Aid Kit.	2. Phone your company's emergency response number or 911 and get the First Aid Kit.	
3. Stop bleeding with pressure.	3. Keep the victim still and calm. Tell the victim not to move the bite area.	
4. Wash the bite area with soap and water under faucet pressure.	4. Gently wash the bite area with soap and water.	
5. It isn't necessary to use a dressing.	5. Do not use a dressing.	5. Apply mild pressure by wrapping elastic bandages over the bite and the entire arm or leg.

You wash the bite gently with water from a hose. You do not know whether the snake was poisonous, but you are told that the snake did not hold on once it struck. So you assume it was not a coral snake. For this reason you do not put a pressure dressing on the bite. You wait with the victim until EMS rescuers arrive.

Insect and Spider Bites and Stings

Case Example

The gardener at your workplace suddenly cries out that a bee has stung her. She asks you to help. She complains that her face feels hot and "tight" and that she has tightness across the chest. She is also having trouble breathing. You notice that her face is red and beginning to look puffy. You hear a whistling noise when she breathes.

Would you know what to do?

Usually insect and spider bites and stings cause only mild pain, itching, and swelling at the bite.

Some insect bites can be serious and even fatal if

- Poison is injected into the victim (for example, a black widow spider or brown recluse spider)
- The victim has a bad allergic reaction to the bite

Actions for Insect and Spider Bites and Stings

1. Make sure that the area is safe for you and the victim.

2. Phone or ask someone to phone your company's emergency response number or 911 and get the First Aid Kit if

    - The victim tells you that he/she has a bad allergic reaction to insect bites
    - The victim has signs of a bad allergic reaction

3. Bees are the only insects that leave their stingers behind. If the victim was stung by a bee, look for the stinger. Scrape away the stinger and venom sac with something hard, such as a credit card, one edge of a pair of scissors, or the back or dull side of a knife. Do not remove the stinger until you make sure that there are no other priorities, such as a bad allergic reaction.

4. Wash the sting or bite area with soap and water.

5. Put an ice bag wrapped in a towel or cloth over the sting or bite area.

6. Watch the victim for at least 30 minutes for signs of a bad allergic reaction (see below).

Signs of a Bad Allergic Reaction

Some people can have a bad allergic reaction to insect bites, especially to bee stings. People who have bad allergic reactions to insect bites often have an epinephrine pen and know how to use it. They often wear medical identification jewelry.

Signs of a bad allergic reaction are

- Swelling of the tongue and face
- Trouble breathing
- Shock

Actions for a Bad Allergic Reaction

1. Phone or ask someone to phone your company's emergency response number (or 911) and get the First Aid Kit.

2. Help the victim get the epinephrine pen and use it if your state and workplace allow you to (see the section on Medical Emergencies).

3. If the victim becomes unresponsive, begin CPR.

4. Do not remove the stinger until there are no signs of the bad allergic reaction.

Case Example (continued)

At the beginning of this section about Insect and Spider Bites and Stings, you read the following Case Example:

The gardener at your workplace suddenly cries out that a bee has stung her. She complains that her face feels hot and "tight" and says that she has tightness across the chest. She is also having trouble breathing. You notice that her face is red and beginning to look puffy. You hear a whistling noise when she breathes.

You read and thought about the following question: Would you know what to do?

Now you know what to do.

You ask the gardener if she has ever had an allergic reaction. She tells you that she is allergic to insect stings and that she has an emergency kit prescribed by her doctor in her car. You tell a co-worker to phone your company's emergency response number and bring the First Aid Kit.

You send another co-worker to get the victim's emergency kit from the victim's car, and you help the gardener to give herself an epinephrine shot. Within minutes the swelling, chest tightness, and wheezing lessen. You take out the stinger and venom sac by scraping the edge of a credit card along the skin. You then wash the area with soap and water and put an ice bag wrapped in a towel over the sting area. You tell the gardener that she is going to be fine.

By the time EMS rescuers arrive, she feels much better. She thanks you. One of the EMS rescuers says, "Nice job. We'll take it from here."

DO NOT

Removing a Bee Stinger

DO NOT pull the stinger out with tweezers or your fingers. Squeezing the venom sac can release more venom.

Poisonous Spiders and Scorpions

The bite of most spiders is so mild that often victims don't even know that they have been bitten. In the United States there are only two spiders and one scorpion whose bite can be fatal for humans. They are

- The black widow spider (see "FYI: Black Widow Spiders" below)
- The brown recluse spider (see "FYI: Brown Recluse Spiders" below)
- The bark scorpion (Figure 3), which is found mainly in the southwestern United States

Signs of Poisonous Spider and Scorpion Bites

The bites of non-poisonous spiders produce mild itching and swelling at the bite. In contrast, the bite from poisonous spiders and scorpions produces general signs. These general signs include the following:

- Muscle cramps
- Headache
- Fever
- Vomiting
- Breathing problems
- Seizures
- Unresponsiveness

Actions for Spider Bites and Scorpion Stings

If signs such as mild pain, swelling, or itching are present only in the bite/sting area:

1. Clean the bite with soap (if available) and water.

2. Put an ice bag over a towel on the bite.

If you know that a victim has been bitten by a poisonous spider or scorpion or if a victim develops general signs:

1. Make sure the area is safe for you and the victim.

2. Phone your company's emergency response number (or 911) immediately and get the First Aid Kit.

3. Wash the bite with soap and water.

4. Put an ice bag wrapped in a towel or cloth on the bite.

5. If the victim becomes unresponsive, begin the steps of CPR.

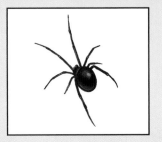
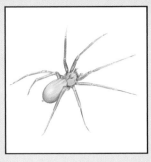
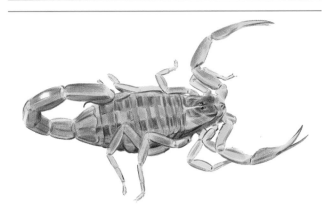

FIGURE 3. Bark scorpion.

Summary of First Aid Actions for Insect Stings and Spider Bites

Bees	Spiders and Scorpions
1. Make sure that the area is safe for you and the victim.	1. Make sure the area is safe for you and the victim.
2. Phone your company's emergency response number or 911 and get the First Aid Kit if the victim has a history or signs of a bad allergic reaction to insects.	2. If the victim was bitten by a poisonous spider or scorpion or has any general signs (see page 102): ■ Phone your company's emergency response number (or 911) and get the First Aid Kit. ■ If the victim becomes unresponsive, begin CPR.
3. Help the victim with medications if signs of a bad allergic reaction appear.	3. Clean the bite or sting area with soap and water.
4. Look for the stinger and remove it. (DO NOT use tweezers or your fingers.)	4. Put an ice bag wrapped in a towel on the bite.
5. Clean the sting area with soap and water.	
6. Put an ice bag wrapped in a towel on the sting area.	
7. Watch the victim for at least 30 minutes for signs of a bad allergic reaction.	

Ticks

Ticks are found in wooded areas. They attach themselves to exposed body parts. Many ticks are harmless. Some carry serious diseases, like Lyme disease. The map, Lyme Disease: Reported Cases (Figure 4), shows the areas in the United States where Lyme disease is likely to occur. Check to see if you live in an area of the country where Lyme disease is common.

If you find a tick (Figure 5), remove it as soon as possible. The longer the tick stays attached to a victim, the greater the victim's chance of catching a disease.

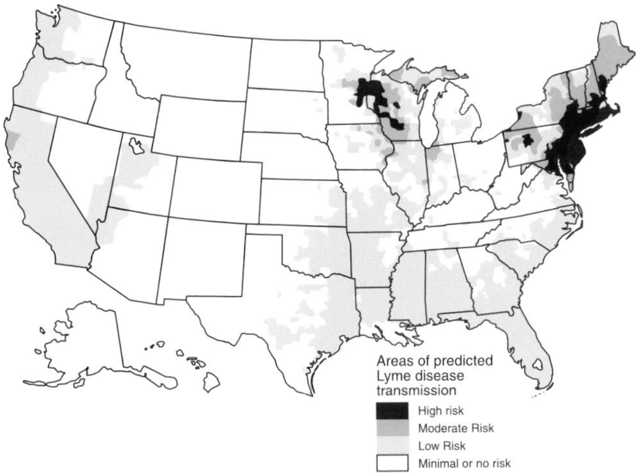

Areas of predicted Lyme disease transmission

■ High risk
▨ Moderate Risk
▧ Low Risk
□ Minimal or no risk

FIGURE 4. Lyme Disease: Reported Cases. Courtesy of the Centers for Disease Control and Prevention.

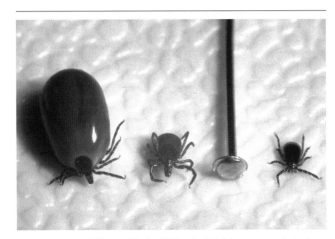

FIGURE 5. Different kinds of ticks. Left tick is engorged; pin is for size. Courtesy of Pfizer Inc.

DO NOT

Wrong Actions for Removing a Tick

The following are the WRONG actions to take when trying to remove a tick:

- **DO NOT** use petroleum jelly.
- **DO NOT** use fingernail polish.
- **DO NOT** use rubbing alcohol.
- **DO NOT** use a hot match.
- **DO NOT** use gasoline.
- **DO NOT** twist or jerk the tick.

Actions for Tick Bites

1. Hold the tick with your fingers (or a special tick-removing tool) as close to the victim's skin as possible. You may use tweezers but try to avoid pinching the tick. Lift the tick straight out without twisting or squeezing its body. If you lift the tick until the skin tents and wait for several seconds, the tick may let go.

2. Wash the bite with soap and water.

3. Put an ice bag wrapped in a towel on the bite.

4. Get medical help if you are in an area where Lyme disease occurs (Figure 4). If possible, place the tick in a plastic bag and give it to the victim.

Review Questions

1. A stray dog has bitten your mail carrier. The man's pants are ripped, and blood is trickling from the upper part of his leg. He asks you for help. Which of the following first aid actions should you perform?

   a. Ask him to lie down and raise his legs about 12 inches

   b. Put ice on the bite

   c. Clean the bite area with soap and water, apply pressure to stop the bleeding, and apply a dressing

   d. Tell him not to worry about it

2. A maintenance worker at your company was cleaning a storage area a few hours ago when he felt something like a sharp pinprick on his arm. He asks you for help because he is sweating and has muscle cramps in his back and cramps in his abdomen. On his arm are 2 tiny red spots with swelling around them. Which of the following first aid actions should you perform?

   a. Put the victim's arm in a sling so it doesn't move

   b. Phone your company's emergency response number and get the First Aid Kit. While you are waiting for help to arrive, clean the wound with soap and water and put an ice bag on it

   c. Scrape away the stinger using a hard object such as the edge of a credit card

   d. Ask him if he has an epinephrine pen and help him with it

3. You are working at a construction site. Your co-worker suddenly screams when a large snake buries its fangs in his arm. You get a quick look at the snake but don't know what kind it is. You and the victim move to a safe place. The victim has 2 fang marks on his arm, and he complains of pain. What should you do?

a. Put an ice bag on the bite immediately

b. Cut the skin between the fang marks with a knife and suck the poison from the wound

c. Suck out the poison with your mouth, being careful not to swallow any

d. Have the victim keep his arm still, keep the victim calm, and phone your worksite's emergency response number

4. An employee at a gardening store asks you for help, saying that a wasp stung her on the neck a half hour ago. She has some pain at the site of the sting but is otherwise well. What should you do?

a. Scrape away the stinger with something hard like the edge of a credit card

b. Reassure the victim that she'll be fine, but phone your company's emergency response number

c. Clean the area and put an ice bag on the sting

d. Ask her if she has an epinephrine pen and help her give herself an injection immediately

How did you do?

1. **The correct answer is c.** The most important immediate actions for animal bites are to clean the wound to reduce the risk of infection and to stop any bleeding.

Answer **a** is incorrect because the victim has no signs of shock, so there is no reason to have him lie down and raise his feet.

Answer **b** is incorrect because putting ice on the wound will not protect the victim from infection and may cause cold injury.

Answer **d** is incorrect because false reassurance is not recommended.

2. **The correct answer is b.** The victim has generalized signs of a bite (muscle cramps and sweating), so you assume that an insect that has injected poison (for example, a black widow spider or brown recluse spider or bark scorpion) has bitten him. You should therefore phone your company's emergency response number and get the First Aid Kit. Clean the bite area while you wait for EMS to arrive.

Answer **a** is incorrect because putting the arm in a sling does nothing helpful for the victim.

Answer **c** is incorrect because bees are the only insects that leave a stinger behind, and these are not signs of a bee sting.

Answer **d** is incorrect because these signs do not indicate a bad allergic reaction.

3. **The correct answer is d.** Although you don't know whether the snake is poisonous, you assume that it is. Tell the victim not to move the arm that was bitten while you phone your company's emergency response number and get the First Aid Kit.

Answer **a** is incorrect because there is no evidence to show that ice slows the absorption of snake poison.

Answers **b** and **c** are incorrect because you should never try to suck poison from a snakebite.

4. **The correct answer is c.** Clean the area and put an ice bag on the sting.

Answer **a** is incorrect because only a bee leaves a stinger; a wasp does not, so there is no stinger to scrape away.

Answers **b** and **d** are incorrect because there are no signs or history of a bad allergic reaction, so there is no reason to phone your company's emergency response number or to give the victim an injection of epinephrine.

Cold-Related Emergencies

Cold-related emergencies may involve only part of the body or the whole body. A cold injury to part of the body is called frostbite. Cold injury to the whole body is called hypothermia.

What You Will Learn

By the end of this chapter you should be able to

- Tell the difference between frostbite and hypothermia
- List the first aid actions for frostbite
- List the first aid actions for hypothermia

Frostbite

Frostbite affects parts of the body that are exposed, such as the fingers, toes, nose, and ears. Frostbite typically occurs outside in cold weather. But it can also occur inside when workers without gloves handle cold materials, such as gases under pressure.

Case Example

You work for a snow removal company. Near the end of your shift your co-worker complains that several fingers of his right hand feel cold and numb. You ask if you can help and you examine his hand. The tips of his right third and fourth fingers feel cold and hard.

Would you know what to do?

Signs of Frostbite

- The skin over the frostbitten area is white, waxy, or grayish-yellow.
- The frostbitten area is cold and numb.
- The frostbitten area is hard, and the skin doesn't move when you push it.

Actions for Frostbite

1. Move the victim to a warm place.

2. Phone or ask someone to phone your company's emergency response number (or 911) and get the First Aid Kit.

3. Remove tight clothing, rings, or bracelets from the frostbitten part.

4. Remove any wet clothing.

5. Do not try to thaw the frozen part if you are close to a medical facility or if you think there may be a chance of refreezing.

DO NOT

Wrong Actions for Treating Frostbite

- **DO NOT** rub or massage the frostbite.
- **DO NOT** use a heating pad, stove, or fire to rewarm a frostbite.
- **DO NOT** give the victim alcohol.
- **DO NOT** give the victim cigarettes.
- **DO NOT** thaw the frozen part if there is any chance of refreezing or if you are close to a medical facility.

Case Example (continued)

At the beginning of this discussion on Cold-Related Emergencies, you read the following Case Example:

You work for a snow removal company. Near the end of your shift your co-worker complains that several fingers of his right hand feel cold and numb. You ask if you can help and you examine his hand. The tips of his right third and fourth fingers feel cold and hard.

You also read and thought about this question: Would you know what to do?

Now you know what to do.

You move the victim to a warm (not hot) place. You phone your company's emergency response plan (or 911) and get the First Aid Kit. You cover the victim with the Mylar blanket to prevent heat loss, but you do not try to thaw the frostbite. The victim is transported to the local hospital. After treatment the victim's frostbite injuries heal.

Hypothermia (Low Body Temperature)

Hypothermia occurs when body temperature falls. Hypothermia is a serious condition that can cause death. A person can develop hypothermia even when the temperature is above freezing.

Case Example

A co-worker has been icing fish on the deck of a fishing boat for more than an hour. He is not wearing cold weather gear. When you find him, he's sitting on the deck and shivering. When you ask if he's OK, he seems confused and does not respond to your question.

Would you know what to do?

Signs of Hypothermia

Signs of hypothermia depend on the victim's body temperature.

- Shivering is present in mild hypothermia but stops when the hypothermia becomes severe.

- The victim may become confused, have a change in personality, be very sleepy, or may be unconcerned about his/her condition.

- Muscles become stiff and rigid and the skin gets ice cold and blue when body temperature drops below 90°F.

- As the victim's body temperature continues to drop, the victim becomes unresponsive, breathing slows, and it may be hard to tell whether the victim is breathing. The victim may appear to be dead.

FYI...

Shivering

- Shivering protects the body by producing heat.

- Shivering stops when body temperature drops below 90°F.

Actions for Hypothermia

1. Get the victim out of the cold.

2. Keep the victim lying flat.

3. Replace wet clothing with dry clothing. Handle the victim gently.

4. Phone or ask someone to phone your company's emergency response number or 911 and get the First Aid Kit.

5. Put blankets, towels, or newspapers under and around the victim, and cover the victim's head but not the face.

6. If the victim is unresponsive, begin CPR.

Case Example (continued)

At the beginning of this discussion about Hypothermia, you read the following Case Example:

A co-worker has been icing fish on the deck of a fishing boat for more than an hour. He is not wearing cold weather gear. When you find him, he's sitting on the deck and shivering. When you ask if he's OK, he seems confused and does not respond to your question.

You read and thought about this question: Would you know what to do?

Now you know what to do.

You bring your co-worker inside the boat and lay him on his back. You gently remove his cold, wet clothing, wrap him in a dry blanket, and cover him, including his head, with additional blankets and the Mylar blanket from the First Aid Kit. You phone your company's emergency response number (or 911) and return to shore for help.

Summary of Cold-Related Injuries

Injury	Signs	Actions
Frostbite	■ The skin over the frostbitten area is white, waxy, or grayish-yellow. ■ The frostbitten area is cold and numb. ■ The frostbitten area is hard, and the skin doesn't move when you push it.	■ Get the victim out of the cold. ■ Keep the victim lying flat. ■ Replace wet clothing with dry clothing. Handle the victim gently. ■ Phone or ask someone to phone your company's emergency response number or 911 and get the First Aid Kit. ■ Put blankets, towels, or newspapers under and around the victim, and cover the victim's head but not the face. ■ If the victim is unresponsive, begin CPR. Do not try to warm the frozen part if you are close to a medical facility or if you think there may be a chance of refreezing.
Hypothermia	■ Shivering is present in mild hypothermia. Shivering stops when the hypothermia becomes severe. ■ The victim may become confused, have a change in personality, be very sleepy, or may be unconcerned about his/her condition. ■ When body temperature drops below 90°F, muscles become stiff and rigid and the skin gets ice cold and blue. ■ As the victim's body temperature continues to drop, the victim becomes unresponsive, breathing slows, and it may be hard to tell whether the victim is breathing. The victim may appear to be dead.	■ Get the victim out of the cold. ■ Keep the victim lying flat. ■ Replace wet clothing with dry clothing. Handle the victim gently. ■ Phone or ask someone to phone your company's emergency response number or 911 and get the First Aid Kit. ■ Put blankets, towels, or newspapers under and around the victim, and cover the victim's head but not the face. ■ If the victim is unresponsive, begin CPR.

Heat-Related Emergencies

Heat-related emergencies result from exposure to extreme heat.

Case Example

On a very hot and humid day a worker for a land-scaping company complains that she feels as if she has the flu. You notice that she is sweating. She complains that she is thirsty, tired, and sick to her stomach and has a headache.

Would you know what to do?

What You Will Learn

By the end of this section you should be able to

- List the signs of a heat-related emergency
- List the signs of heatstroke
- List the first aid actions for a heat-related emergency
- List the first aid actions for heatstroke

Signs of Heat-Related Emergencies

Heat-related emergencies range in severity from mild to life-threatening. We will call the life-threatening signs of a heat related emergency "heatstroke." You must recognize and give first aid for heat-related emergencies early because someone with mild signs can get worse quickly and develop heatstroke.

Many of the signs of a heat-related emergency are similar to those of the flu. So people with a heat-related emergency sometimes think that they are developing flu.

The signs of a heat-related emergency are

- Muscle cramps
- Sweating
- Headache
- Nausea
- Weakness
- Dizziness

The signs of heatstroke are

- Confusion or strange behavior
- Inability to drink or vomiting
- Red, hot, and dry skin (the victim may stop sweating)
- Shallow breathing, seizures, or unresponsiveness

Critical Facts

Don't Ignore Heat-Related Warning Signs

Symptoms of heat-related emergencies often get worse if left untreated. Mild heat-related signs are a warning that the victim may develop heatstroke unless you take action!

Actions for Heat-Related Emergencies

1. Move the victim to a cool or shady area.
2. Loosen or remove tight clothing.
3. Encourage the victim to drink water.
4. Sponge or spray the victim with cool *(not ice-cold)* water and fan the victim.
5. Phone or ask someone to phone your company's emergency response number immediately if there are any signs of heatstroke, and continue to cool the victim until rescuers arrive.
6. If the victim becomes unresponsive, phone 911 and start CPR as needed.

DO NOT

Wrong Actions for Treating Heat-Related Injuries

- **DO NOT** wait to begin cooling the victim until EMS rescuers arrive. Every minute counts!
- **DO NOT** continue cooling after the victim's mental state has improved. Unnecessary cooling could lead to hypothermia.
- **DO NOT** use rubbing alcohol to cool the victim.
- **DO NOT** give the victim anything to drink or eat if the victim cannot swallow or is vomiting.

Case Example (continued)

At the beginning of this discussion about Heat-Related Emergencies, you read the following Case Example:

On a very hot and humid day a worker for a landscaping company complains that she feels as if she has the flu. You notice that she is sweating. She complains that she is thirsty, tired, and sick to her stomach and has a headache.

You read this question: Would you know what to do?

Now you know what to do.

The worker wants to finish the job, but you insist that she stop and rest in a shady area. You sponge her face, chest, arms, and legs with cool water while you fan her. Within 20 minutes she feels much better.

Summary of Signs of and First Aid Actions for Heat-Related Emergencies

Signs	Actions
Heat-Related Emergency ■ Muscle cramps ■ Sweating ■ Headache ■ Nausea ■ Weakness ■ Dizziness	■ Move the victim to a cool or shady area. ■ Loosen or remove tight clothing. ■ Encourage the victim to drink water. ■ Sponge or spray the victim with cool (*not ice cold*) water and fan the victim. ■ Phone or ask someone to phone your company's emergency response number immediately if there are any signs of heatstroke, and continue to cool the victim until rescuers arrive. ■ If the victim becomes unresponsive, phone 911 and start CPR as needed.
Heatstroke ■ Confusion or strange behavior ■ Inability to drink or vomiting ■ Red, hot, and dry skin (the victim may stop sweating) ■ Shallow breathing, seizures, or unresponsiveness	■ Phone or ask someone to phone your company's emergency response number or 911. ■ Move the victim to a cool or shady area. ■ Loosen or remove tight clothing. ■ Encourage the victim to drink water if the victim is not vomiting. ■ Sponge or spray the victim with cool (*not ice cold*) water and fan the victim. ■ If the victim becomes unresponsive, start CPR as needed. Move the victim to a cool or shady area.

Review Questions

1. **It's winter at a construction site. Your co-worker has frostbite on the fingertips of one hand. A medical facility is about 15 minutes away. Which of the following is the best first aid to provide?**

   a. Rub the fingertips for several minutes to warm them

   b. Put a chemical heat pack on the fingertips

   c. Move the co-worker to a warm place and phone your company's emergency response number or 911

   d. Rapidly rewarm the fingertips in warm water

2. **A 26-year-old man has fallen through the ice covering a pond at your workplace. Several bystanders pull him from the water. He is responsive and shivering. Someone has already phoned your company's emergency response number and the EMS system and has brought the First Aid Kit. You are a designated First Aid rescuer. Which of the following first aid actions would be best for you to perform until EMS rescuers arrive?**

   a. Do nothing until EMS rescuers arrive

   b. Get the victim out of the cold, help him change into dry clothing, and wrap his head and body with any available covering or with the Mylar blanket from the First Aid Kit

   c. Cover the victim with a blanket but leave all of his clothing in place; do not move him at all

   d. Tell the victim to exercise vigorously to keep warm until the EMS responders arrive

3. **While working at a construction site on a hot summer day, your co-worker suddenly falls on one knee and complains of a bad cramp in the muscle of his leg. He has no other complaints and seems completely responsive. He asks for your help. Which of the following first aid actions should you perform?**

   a. Phone your company's emergency response number and get the First Aid Kit; then move the victim to a cool spot; have him loosen or remove some of his clothes; then spray him with water and fan him

   b. Move the victim to a cool spot; have him loosen or remove some of his clothes; spray him with water and fan him; and phone your company's emergency response number or 911

   c. Have him rest in a cool spot, drink water, and loosen or remove tight clothing

   d. Have him rest in a cool spot; raise his legs and dry his skin with a towel

4. **While working outside on a very hot and humid day, a co-worker complains that she feels sick to her stomach, has a headache, and is very tired. She is very sweaty. Which of the following actions would be best for you to perform to help this co-worker now?**

   a. Phone your company's emergency response number, move the victim to a cool spot, remove as much of her clothing as possible, spray her with water, and fan her

   b. Move her to a cool spot, remove as much of her clothing as possible, spray her with water, fan her, and phone your company's emergency response number

   c. Have her rest in a cool spot and drink water

   d. Have her rest in a cool spot, raise her legs, and use a towel to dry her skin

5. **Your company is sponsoring a marathon race on a very hot day. You are giving first aid at the race. One of the runners drops to the ground. She is confused and makes no sense. Her skin is very hot to the touch.**

Which of the following first aid actions should you perform?

  a. Phone your company's emergency response number immediately, then move the runner to a cool spot, remove as much of her clothing as possible, spray her with water, and fan her

  b. Move the runner to a cool spot, remove as much of her clothing as possible, spray her with water, and fan her

  c. Have the runner rest in a cool spot and have her drink lots of water

  d. Have the runner rest in a cool spot, raise her legs, and dry her skin with a towel

How did you do?

1. **The correct answer is c.** Frostbite is a serious problem. You should immediately move the victim to a warm place and phone your company's emergency response number.

Answer **a** is incorrect because you should never rub a body part that is frostbitten because it can damage the frozen tissue.

Answers **b** and **d** are incorrect because you should leave the rewarming of a body part to a medical facility if such a facility is nearby.

2. **The correct answer is b.** The victim is already cold (shivering). He can become hypothermic unless you move him to a warm place, have him change from his wet clothes into dry clothes, and wrap him in blankets, newspapers, or anything that will save body heat. You should also phone your company's emergency response number and get the First Aid Kit. You may use the Mylar blanket from the First Aid Kit to help warm the victim.

Answer **a** is incorrect because waiting for EMS wastes valuable time during which the victim will become colder.

Answers **c** and **d** are incorrect because covering the victim without removing wet clothing

and without bringing the victim out of the cold is useless, as is exercise.

3. **The correct answer is c.** Muscle cramps are a sign of heat-related injury. At this point the signs are mild, so you only need to tell the victim to rest in a cool place, drink water, and loosen tight clothing.

Answers **a** and **b** are incorrect because the victim seems to have no signs of a bad heat-related emergency (heatstroke), so there is no reason to phone your company's emergency response number at this time.

Answer **d** is incorrect because the victim is not in shock and therefore there is no need to raise his legs.

4. **The correct answer is c.** Have the victim rest in a cool place and drink water. If she vomits the water, then you would need to phone your company's emergency response number. This victim has more serious signs of heat-related injury than the victim in question 3, but she does not yet have the signs of a bad heat-related emergency (heatstroke). For this reason answers **a** and **b** are incorrect.

Answer **d** is incorrect because the victim has no signs of shock, so there is no reason to raise her legs.

5. **The correct answer is a.** This victim has confusion, a sign of a bad heat-related emergency (heatstroke). You should phone your company's emergency response number before you do anything else. You should then help to cool the victim and monitor the victim's responsiveness closely. If she becomes unresponsive, prepare to support her with CPR if needed.

Answers **b** and **c** are incorrect because you should get help for the victim *before* you begin cooling her.

Answer **d** is incorrect because the victim is not in shock and there is no need to raise her legs.

C h a p t e r ③ *Poison Emergencies*

Poisons

According to the American Association of Poison Centers, a poison is anything someone swallows, breathes, or gets in the eyes or on the skin that causes sickness or death. Many products can poison people. This chapter will not deal with specific poisons. It will deal with general principles of first aid for a poisoning victim. Follow your workplace guidelines about poisonous products in your workplace.

Case Example

You work in an electronics assembly plant. You see a co-worker coughing and rubbing her eyes. She tells you that she has just splashed a cleaning liquid on her face and asks if you will help her.

Would you know what to do?

What You Will Learn

By the end of this chapter you should be able to

■ Recognize the signs of poisoning

■ Know where to find more information about the poison

■ Be able to perform first aid actions quickly and safely

Actions for Poison Emergencies

If you think that someone may have been exposed to a poison:

1. Phone or ask someone to phone your company's emergency response number (or 911) and get the First Aid Kit.

2. Make sure the area is safe before you approach the victim. If the area seems unsafe, do not enter. Tell everyone to move away from the area.

■ Look for signs that warn you that poisons are nearby (Figure 6).

■ Look out for spilled or leaking bottles or boxes.

■ Do not enter the area if you see more than one poisoning victim.

■ Before you approach the victim, put on appropriate protective equipment (mask, gloves, goggles, and suit).

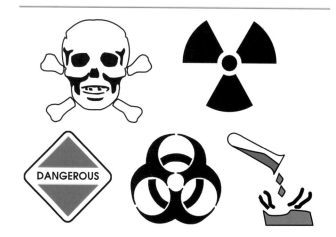

FIGURE 6. Look for warning signs of poisons nearby.

3. Try to move the victim from the area of the poison if you can do so safely. Ask everyone to move away from the area.

■ Help the victim to go outdoors or move to an area of fresh air if possible.

4. If a victim is unresponsive, begin CPR, but do not perform mouth-to-mouth breathing if the poison has contaminated the victim's lips or mouth. Use a barrier device such as a breathing mask.

5. Wash or remove the poison from the victim's skin and clothing if you can do so safely.

■ Help the victim to a safety shower or eye wash station if the victim is responsive and can move (Figure 7).

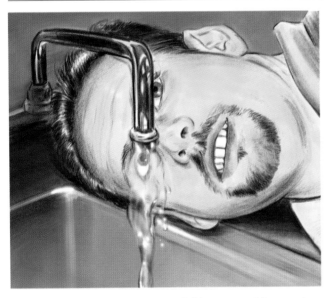

FIGURE 7. Help the victim wash his eyes and face under a sink or an eye wash station.

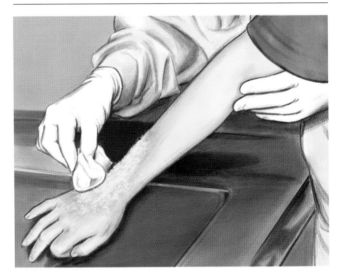

FIGURE 8. Brush off any dry powder or solid substances from the victim's skin with your gloved hand.

- Help the victim take off contaminated clothing and jewelry, with permission.

- Brush off any dry powder or solid substances from the victim's skin with your gloved hand (Figure 8).

- Run water over the skin, eyes, and other contaminated areas of the victim's body for at least 20 minutes or until EMS rescuers arrive. Ask the victim to blink as much as possible while rinsing his/her eyes.

6. If you can identify the poison, send someone to get the MSDS.

- Worksites should have an MSDS (Material Safety Data Sheet) for each poison at the worksite. You should know where the MSDS is at your worksite. The MSDS provides a description of how a specific poison can be harmful. This information can be very helpful at the worksite. It can also be useful to poison centers for identifying a poison and its effects. Unfortunately the MSDS usually provides little information about first aid actions. According to the American Association of Poison centers, some of the first aid actions listed in the MSDS or on the label of the poison may be outdated. You will probably receive additional training on the MSDS during the "Right to Know" training your workplace provides.

7. When you know the name of the poison, call the nearest poison center for instructions on giving first aid. The local poison centers can help you deal with poisons. You should keep the telephone number of the nearest poison center in your First Aid Kit. To contact the nearest poison center:

- Check the front cover of the phone book for the telephone number, or go to the following website: www.aapcc.org.

- In many communities the 911 dispatcher can connect you with the local poison center.

- Phone 800-222-1222. This will connect you to the nearest poison center. Write the number of the nearest poison center with the other emergency telephone numbers on your First Aid Kit.

Case Example (continued)

At the beginning of this chapter about Poisoning Emergencies, you read the following Case Example:

You work in an electronics assembly plant. You see a co-worker coughing and rubbing her eyes. She tells you that she has just splashed a cleaning liquid on her face and asks if you will help her.

You read this question: *Would you know what to do?*

Now you know what to do.

You help the co-worker to a safety shower. She washes the chemical from her face. You send a co-worker to phone your company's emergency response number and get the First Aid Kit. The plant safety professional comes to help. She has the material safety data sheet (MSDS) for the cleaning liquid. She calls the local poison center for advice on first aid actions. When EMS rescuers arrive, you give them the MSDS and information from the poison center.

DO NOT

Wrong Actions for a Poisoning Injury

- **DO NOT** give the victim anything by mouth unless you have been told to do so by trained medical personnel or the poison center.
- **DO NOT** rely on only the first aid instructions on the label of the bottle, can, or box.
- **DO NOT** apply any ointments or lotions to the skin.

FYI...

Calling the Poison Center

When you call the poison center, try to have the following information ready:

- What is the name of the poison? Can you describe it if you cannot name it?
- How much poison did the victim touch, breathe, or swallow?
- About how old is the victim? What is the victim's approximate weight?
- When did the poisoning happen?
- How is the victim feeling or acting now?

Appendix
General Groups of Poisons

The following table lists general groups of poisons and other possibly dangerous substances with information on how the substance may enter the body. This information is for reference only. It does not include all possible classifications or examples of poisonous substances. The first aid rescuer is not expected to know all of these from memory.

Classification	Examples of Dangerous Substances and Methods of Entry into the Body	
Plants	Mistletoe (S) Poinsettias and holly (S) Dieffenbachia (S) Foxglove (S)	Poison ivy (T, S) Poison sumac (T, S) Poison oak (T, S) Philodendron (S)
Gases	Carbon monoxide (B) Propane (B)	Methane and natural gas (B)
Corrosives/acids	Pool cleaner (B, T) Metal-cleaning solution (B, T)	Chlorine (B, T) Ammonia (B, T)
Hydrocarbons	Enamel paint (B, S) Diesel fuel or gasoline (B, T, S)	Lighter fluid (B, T, S) Turpentine (B, T, S)
Household products	Drain cleaners (B, S, T) Oven cleaners (B, S, T) Toilet bowl cleaners (B, S, T) Disinfectants (B, S, T) Laundry detergents (S, T) Bleach (S, B, T) Pesticides and insecticides (S, B, T)	Alcoholic beverages (S) Rubbing alcohol (S, T) Furniture polish (S, T) Gasoline, kerosene (S, B, T) Antifreeze (S, T) Windshield cleaner (S, T)
Personal care products	Mouthwash (S) Perfume and cologne (S, T)	Nail polish and polish remover (S, B, T)
Medicines/ vitamins	Nonprescription medicines, including aspirin, acetaminophen, antacids, laxatives, vitamins (S)	Prescription medicines (S)
Other chemicals	Glues and adhesives (S, B, T) Soldering flux (S, B, T)	

S indicates swallowed; B, breathed; and T, touched.

Review Questions

1. **Your co-worker tells you that her arms are burning. You notice that her shirt and arms are wet with a chemical she uses in her job. You note that she is able to walk without difficulty. Which of the following first aid actions should you perform *first*?**

   a. Take her to the nearest phone, and phone your company's emergency response number

   b. Take her to the plant medical facility

   c. Tell her to go home and take a bath

   d. Take her to the nearest safety shower to wash off the chemical

2. **Your co-worker asks you for help when several people are poisoned by a gas leak in a nearby room. As you approach the area, you see that several people are having trouble breathing. You also see 2 people lying on the floor. They do not appear to be moving. Another co-worker has phoned your company's emergency response number, and EMS responders are on their way. While you wait for help, which of the following should you do *first*?**

   a. Encourage victims who can walk to leave the room and move to an area of fresh air

   b. Enter the room to remove the victims

   c. Enter the room and begin CPR for the people lying on the floor

   d. Get the MSDS for the gas

3. **A co-worker shouts for help. She says she splashed nail polish remover into her eyes. Her eyes are burning. Another co-worker has phoned your company's emergency response number. Which of the following is the best action for you to take *first*?**

   a. Bandage both of the victim's eyes and wait for help to arrive

   b. Have the victim flush her eyes and face with water for at least 20 minutes while she blinks frequently

   c. Phone the poison center for first aid instructions

   d. Review the MSDS for a possible antidote

How did you do?

1. **The correct answer is d.** If you can do so safely, wash off any poison on the victim's skin.

   Answers **a, b**, and **c** are incorrect because they waste time before the poison is washed off.

2. **The correct answer is a.** You should encourage people who can leave the room to do so.

   Answers **b** and **c** are incorrect because you should not put yourself in danger by entering a room where two or more people have been poisoned.

   Answer **d** is incorrect because getting the MSDS is important but not as important as getting the victims to a safer area.

3. **The correct answer is b.** Your first action should be to get rid of as much of the poison as possible by having the victim flush her eyes and face with running water for at least 20 minutes.

   Answer **a** is incorrect because bandaging the eyes traps the poison in the eyes and will do more harm.

   Answers **c** and **d** are incorrect. Phoning the poison center and reviewing the MSDS are both important, but your *first* priority is to prevent more harm.

Environmental Emergencies

Index